HIV and AIDS in Darjeeling

ABOUT THE AUTHOR

Binu Sundas, is an Assistant Professor in the Department of Social Systems and Anthropology, Sikkim University and is currently the Department Co-ordinator. He is the founding member of the department. He completed his Ph.D from Jawaharlal Nehru University, New Delhi. He is a native of Kurseong, District Darjeeling and is a Goethals' Alumni. His area of research interest has been sociology of health. For his M.Phil dissertation he has worked on *"Alcohol Consumption and Health of the People in Darjeeling Hills: An Analysis of Socio-Cultural and Development Factor."* He has done exclusive research in the hills of Darjeeling.

Before joining Sikkim University he worked as a consultant in Educational Development North East Region Unit, IGNOU, New Delhi. He has also written units on tribes of UP and Delhi for IGNOU's Post Graduate Diploma in Social Work. He has also worked as a researcher with Action Aid International, New Delhi and was part of the team writing the report 'Time to Act II: Positive Voices: Emerging Governance Issues on HIV and AIDS in Asia'. He has also worked with Indian Institute of Dalit studies as a researcher for the project, 'Dalit Children and their Discrimination in Various Dimensions.'

HIV and AIDS in DARJEELING

Emerging Socio-Political Challenge

Binu Sundas

CONCEPT PUBLISHING COMPANY PVT. LTD.,
NEW DELHI-110059

ISBN-13: 978-81-8069-815-6

First Published 2011

Published and Printed by

Concept
Since 1974

Concept Publishing Company Pvt. Ltd.
Regd. Office:
A/15-16, Commercial Block, Mohan Garden,
New Delhi-110059 (INDIA)
Phones : 25351460, 25351794, *Fax* : 091-11-25357109
Email : publishing@conceptpub.com,
Website: www.conceptpub.com

Editorial Office:
H-13, Bali Nagar, New Delhi-110 015, India.

Cataloging in Publication Data--*Courtesy:* D.K. Agencies (P) Ltd. <docinfo@dkagencies.com>

Sundas, Binu.
HIV and AIDS in Darjeeling : emerging socio-political challenge / Binu Sundas.
p. cm.
Includes bibliographical references (p.) and index.
ISBN 9788180698156

1. HIV infections—Social aspects—India—Darjeeling. 2. AIDS (Disease)—Social aspects—India—Darjeeling. 3. Darjeeling (India)—Population—Health aspects. 4. Medical policy—India—Darjeeling. I. Title. II. Title: Human immunodeficiency virus and acquired immuno-deficiency syndrome in Darjeeling.

DDC 362.19697920095414 23

Preface

Human Immunodeficiency Virus (HIV) and Acquired Immunodeficiency Syndrome (AIDS) pose a great threat to the human population as has no other epidemics in the history of mankind. HIV/AIDS was identified only in the early 1980s in the USA. HIV/AIDS is affecting most of the regions in the world and is posing tremendous challenge to the civil society and Government. It has in a single stroke destroyed the developmental gains made in years. HIV/AIDS epidemic has continued to grow and this growth has been facilitated by the globalizing world, with faster means of communication and constant movement of the people. When sexual intercourse and sharing of needles among the intravenous drug users were recognized as the primary modes of transmission, it was observed that the high risk groups like the commercial sex workers, their clients and the intravenous drug users were more vulnerable and susceptible to infection. However, with time HIV/AIDS has made inroads into our social spaces and has rendered vulnerable each and every individual, ranging from the high risk groups to the house wives.

HIV/AIDS is not just a medical issue but it is rooted in the social, economic, political and cultural context and poverty, migration, gender inequality, access to health services all play a pertinent role in the spread of HIV/AIDS. In India a large proportion of the population are still in poverty and migrate from one part of the country to another in search of livelihood. In such cases they may engage themselves in activities which are conducive to the spread of HIV/AIDS. The patriarchal nature of the Indian society also facilitates the spread of HIV/AIDS. The women, especially the wives, do not have any say in the domestic life and regarding sexual matters they are at the mercy of their husbands which puts them in greater risk contracting HIV/AIDS. The absence of condom use among the consenting couples also poses a great threat to the women.

The first case of HIV infection in India was detected among the sex workers of Chennai and was subsequently reported from brothels from other parts of country. In the North East India HIV infection was reported from among the intravenous drug users and their partners. The pattern of HIV infection in India is as diverse as the country itself. In a relatively short span of time the virus has spread to different parts of the country.

The first case of infection in Darjeeling was identified in the year 2002. In five years time the number of people infected had reached 141. The absence of a stable political situation and the lack of employment opportunities had forced many to migrate to other parts of the country and this has also facilitated the growth of HIV infection in the region. The absence of proper medical facilities and the lack of awareness among the people with regards to HIV/AIDS is also a cause of worry in the hills of Darjeeling. The lack of financial help to the NGOs is also a hindrance towards the prevention and control activities. Amidst the constraints Shanker Foundation has been able to help the PLWHAs to fight the stigma and discrimination associated with the disease.

Shanker Foundation is the most prominent among all the NGOs confronting the virus in the hills of Darjeeling. The Foundation works for the betterment of all the PLWHAs of the hills under enormous constraints and its single most important strength has been its ability to improve the quality of life of its members. However, there are other indicators that show success of a different kind. An important indictor has been the Foundation's ability to attract volunteers who do not have a direct stake in HIV/AIDS. For instance, in addition to the PLWHAs and their relatives, the Foundation has attracted the participation of a number of volunteers who are not sero positive and have no family members living with the virus. However, the work of Shanker Foundation has been handicapped by the lack of support from the civil society and the stigma and discrimination and most importantly the reluctance of members to disclose their positive status.

This book is developed from my Ph.D thesis titled 'HIV/AIDS in Darjeeling: An Analysis of Population Dynamics and Institutional Response' with few addition and deletion here and there. The introductory chapter highlights the crisis of HIV/AIDS and also focuses on the methodology. It also identifies the issues associated with HIV/AIDS with the help of a comprehensive review of literature on HIV/AIDS. The socio-political history of Darjeeling, in a brief manner is dealt with in the second chapter to substantiate the later arguements and also discusses the risk factors associated with HIV/AIDS and prevalence in the study area. Shanker Foundation is also discussed in the chapter.

The third chapter deals with the socio demographic conditions of the sample population and also analyses in detail each category of the groups of people that make up the sample population. The chapter profiles the PLWHA and highlights their various experiences. The fourth chapter deals with mobility, sexual behaviour and trends among the people, risk groups, the knowledge and perception of HIV/AIDS among the people and also the stigma and discrimination associated with HIV/AIDS in the hills of Darjeeling. The fifth chapter gives a brief account of international response to HIV/AIDS and primarily focuses on the responses from various institutions in the hills of Darjeeling, to control and prevent the epidemic.

The sixth chapter discusses the spread of HIV/AIDS through population mobility, use of technology, substance abuse, sexual behaviour, knowledge and experiences of the infected and affected persons. The chapter also illustrates the findings and proposes some strategies to address the epidemic in Darjeeling hills. The concluding chapter summarizes the thesis and on the basis of the thesis draws conclusions.

Acknowledgements

I take this opportunity to thank my mentor and supervisor during my M.Phil/Ph.D programme, Dr. Sanghmitra Acharya who always extended constant support and advice during the course of my dissertation and since my first year in M.Phil. She has been a constant source of inspiration to me as she epitomizes hard work and sincerity in all her efforts. More than being a good teacher she has been a person of high quality which has inspired me in my endeavour. She has shown immense patience with me all these years. The Center of Social Medicine & Community Health (JNU) deserves a special mention as it has played an important role in shaping up my perspective regarding the health of the people. Coming to this center for the M.Phil/Ph.D programme was an eye opener for me with regards to the understanding of health. I am also grateful to the teachers of the centre for al: the support and encouragement they have had for me.

I take this opportunity to show my gratitude to my parents. They have been the best possible parents. They have been very selfless in supporting me. They have always installed in me the value of education. I hope this work reflects the inspiration I got from them.

There have been many people who have provided me with the opportunity think about HIV/AIDS and I am indebted to all of them. Hari and Polsen from the Shanker Foundation had been very kind to help me establish contacts with all the people concerned with HIV/AIDS in Darjeeling hills. If it were not for them then this work would have never completed. I am very thankful to them and all the respondents who shared with me their opinions regarding HIV/AIDS as well as the 'Person Living With HIV/AIDS who were willing to share with me their experiences of being infected by the virus and all the ordeals they have to undergo.

I am also thankful to Bidhya didi, Bibu, Anu dada and Lokesh for their love and encouragement. I am also very grateful to the rest of my family members for their love and support. All my friends whose names if I write will fill more than a few pages have also been a constant source of encouragement to me and I am thankful to them.

I am forever indebted to my wife for all the help she has provided. She also read the first and second draft and made extensive comments, making many useful and constructive suggestions which I have tried to include as expansively as possible. She has been instrumental in the completion of this work.

I am also grateful to the library staff of all the libraries I have used for the completion of this work. Last but not the least I am thankful to all the NGOs in Darjeeling district and also the respondents who were willing to share with me whatever they knew about HIV/AIDS. I am also grateful to the doctors in Kurseong sub divisional hospital, Kalimpong sub divisional hospital and Darjeeling *'sadar'* hospital.

Binu Sundas

Contents

Chapter I

HIV/AIDS in Darjeeling: A Cause for Concern

Background

The HIV/AIDS epidemic is one of the greatest humanitarian crises of all times. It is destroying the lives and livelihoods of millions of people around the world. It causes death and untold misery, destroys families and communities. It breaks the social norms and values of the society (Nelkin *et al.* 1991) and it is a vicious cycle which affects directly or indirectly every individual in a society. It has had tremendous impact on the development gains of several years and in a single stroke has ruptured the social fabric of the society. It is a source of enormous psycho-social, mental and physical stress to individuals who are infected as well as affected by it. That is why it has become a salient component in the agenda of health personnels across the world, and has received unprecedented attention. At present, there is no vaccine or drug to cure it and scholars like Kalichman (1998) think that even if a cure were to be found it will be so expensive that it would not be universally accessible. In the absence of vaccines and drugs to combat HIV/AIDS, a greater responsibility has been placed in the hands of human service professionals caring for People Living with HIV/AIDS (PLWHA) who has to confront many challenges resulting from HIV/AIDS infection—social, economic, lack of knowledge and shortage of trained medical staff.

The origin of HIV/AIDS has puzzled scientists as well as

the public ever since the disease first came to light in the early 1980s. Since then it has been a subject of debates and a broad range of theories regarding its origin have emerged. These theories however do not converge to a common point but gives diverse perspective on the origin and spread of HIV/AIDS. It is unlikely that the truth regarding how, when and where HIV/AIDS actually originated will be known. A combination of many factors have attributed to the spread of the virus and undoubtedly certain features of the 20th century, like faster means of travel, communication and drug abuse etc. have played a major role in its global spread.

Regarding the origin of HIV/AIDS, there are three prevalent thoughts. One is that HIV was well established in all areas of the world but has only recently been recognized. However, this theory has not been well substantiated. A second proposition holds that HIV evolved through mutation of an older and non-pathogenic virus. Virologists however, have dismissed this explanation for HIV on the basis of specific characteristics of the virus and its relationship to other viruses. A third and widely discussed possible origin of HIV is zoonosis—the transmission of a non-human virus into human population. Zoonosis is the probable explanation for HIV because similar viruses exist in apes of Africa where HIV is endemic (Goudsmit 1997). However, the most widely held view is that a virus developed in humans in Central Africa and only recently spread to other regions of the world, primarily through global travel and transcontinental commerce has caused HIV to originate (Kalichman 1998). Epidemiological data provide the strongest support for this theory.

HIV/AIDS—The Global Scenario

In June 1981, the Centre for Disease Control in the United States of America reported the first clinical evidence of AIDS (Muthuswamy 2005). It was then an epidemic of the urban gay population and was called a 'gay related immune disease' (Lorber 1997). However, it has moved from being a 'gay disease' to affect individuals across regions, race, sex, ethnicities and is becoming 'more complex every year' (McKee *et al.* 2004).

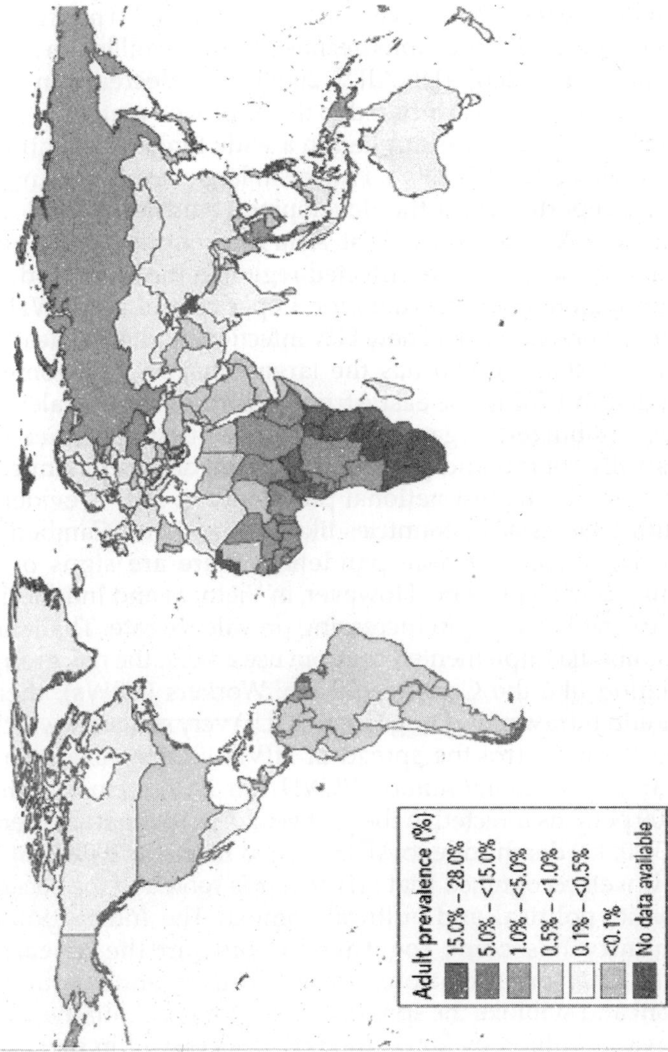

Map 1.1: Prevalence of HIV/AIDS among Adults in Different Countries, 2007

Source: 2008 Report on the Global AIDS Epidemic.

In the last two decades the epidemic has spread all-over the world. Countries in southern Africa have the highest prevalence ranging between 15-20 per cent. Nordic countries have prevalence below 1 per cent (Map 1.1). Globally over 33 million people were living with HIV/AIDS in 2007. The annual number of new HIV infections declined from 3.0 million in 2001 to 2.7 million in 2007 (UNAIDS 2008). This decrease in the number of PLWHA is attributed to the improved methodology of estimation which was applied to a wide range of countries in the world (UNAIDS 2007). However, large numbers of new cases are reported from the developing countries, mainly in Sub-Sahara Africa, South-East Asia and South Asia. Sub-Saharan Africa is the most affected region in the world today. The sub-region alone accounts for 35 per cent of all PLWHA and almost one-third of all new HIV infections and AIDS deaths globally in 2007. It also has the largest majority of women infected with HIV. In the east African countries the prevalence rate has stabilized. Uganda is one of the first countries to successfully control and prevent the spread of the epidemic.

In Asia the highest national prevalence of HIV is evident in South-East Asia. In countries like Thailand and Cambodia where HIV/AIDS became pandemic, there are signs of a declining prevalence rate. However, in Vietnam and Indonesia there are evidences of an increasing prevalence rate. Thailand and Cambodia implemented condom use among the risk group population like the Commercial Sex Workers (CSWs), their clients and Intravenous Drug Users (IDUs) very seriously which helped them control the spread of HIV/AIDS. In Asia, there were an estimated 4.9 million PLWHA in 2007, including the 4,40,000 persons infected in the past year. Approximately, there were 3,00,000 deaths due to AIDS-related illness in 2007 (*Ibid.*).

It is well recognized that HIV/AIDS is rooted in the social, economic, political and cultural context. The International community has come together to confront the disease. International organizations are making an endeavour to confront and stabilize the spread of the epidemic. Initiative like the 'Treat 3 Million by 2005,' though unsuccessful in meeting the target, was introduced. Now the G8 leaders have pledged a new goal of coming as close as possible to universal AIDS treatment access by 2010. Different governments have formulated different policies to combat the disease. However, the efficacy of such policies is determined by the degree of governance and a presence of a functional civil society. Good governance is the key to development and success of policies which are essential to address the HIV/AIDS epidemic. Political stability and the participation of civil society are prominent determinants for the effectiveness of governance. However, social stigma and discrimination associated with HIV/AIDS and inadequate public health systems severely impedes the implementation of the policies like availability and delivery of effective interventions such as prevention, education, risk reduction counselling, condom distribution and needle exchange programmes.

HIV/AIDS in India

In India, HIV infection was first reported from among the sex workers in Chennai in 1986 and immediately thereafter it was found among the CSWs of Mumbai. Since then the virus has unprecedentedly spread to other parts of the country. In 1987, a National AIDS Control Programme was launched to co-ordinate national responses. Its activities covered surveillance, blood screening, and health education (NACO 2005). By the end of 1987, out of 52,907 who had been tested, around 135 people were found to be HIV positive and 14 had AIDS (Kakar and Kakar 2001). Most of these initial cases had occurred through heterosexual sex, but by the end of the 1980s, a rapid spread of HIV was observed among IDUs in Manipur, Mizoram and Nagaland—three north-eastern states of India bordering Myanmar (Panda 2002). Drugs from Myanmar come to these states as the border is not properly guarded and also because of insurgency. The drugs from these states are further trafficked to Siliguri, which can be reached within less than 48 hours. Once the drugs reach Siliguri it easily reaches Darjeeling. Today in India the number of PLWHA is very high, representing a tremendous public health burden. The HIV affliction levels among High Risk Groups (HRGs) are being closely monitored all-over the country. The proportion of population infected has crossed one per cent in six states. These states are Maharashtra, Karnataka, Tamil Nadu, Andhra Pradesh, Manipur and

Nagaland and are termed as high prevalence states and account for 75 per cent of the country's estimated HIV/AIDS cases. Increase in numbers of HIV positive cases is being noticed in states of Rajasthan, West Bengal, Gujarat, Bihar and Madhya Pradesh. Although, the recent data has revealed that HIV prevalence has stabilized in Tamil Nadu, Andhra Pradesh, Karnataka, and Maharashtra, it is increasing in at-risk populations in other states such as West Bengal, Gujarat. In 2008, the figure was confirmed to be 2.5 million which equates to a prevalence of 0.3 per cent (UNAIDS 2008). While this rate may seem low, as India's total population is very high, this translates into a high volume of PLWHA. With a population of more than a billion, a mere 0.1 per cent increase in HIV prevalence would increase the estimated number of PLWHA by over half a million.

Based on the women attending Ante Natal Clinic (ANC) prevalence, the states and Union Territories are broadly divided into the high, moderate and low prevalence categories. There are inter-state and intra-state diversity, in the pattern of HIV transmission. There is a wide variance in HIV prevalence between districts and intra-districts as is evident from the sentinel surveillance data. Based on these data, the districts have also been categorized as A, B, C, D. The district which has been categorized as A indicates more than 1 per cent ANC/PPTCT (Prevention of Parent to Child Transmission) prevalence in district in any time in any of the site in the last 3 years. The district which has been categorized as B indicates less than 1 per cent ANC/PPCTC prevalence in all the sites during last 3 years associated with more than 5 per cent prevalence in any HRG group (CSW/MSM/IDU). The district which has been categorized as C indicates less than 1 per cent in ANC prevalence in all sites during last 3 years with less than 5 per cent in all STD clinic attendees or any HRG with known hot spots (Migrants, truckers, large aggregation of factory workers etc.). The district which has been categorized as D indicates less than 1 per cent ANC prevalence in all sites during last 3 years with less than 5 per cent in all STD attendees or any HRG or no or poor HIV data with no known hot spots/unknown (NACO 2006).

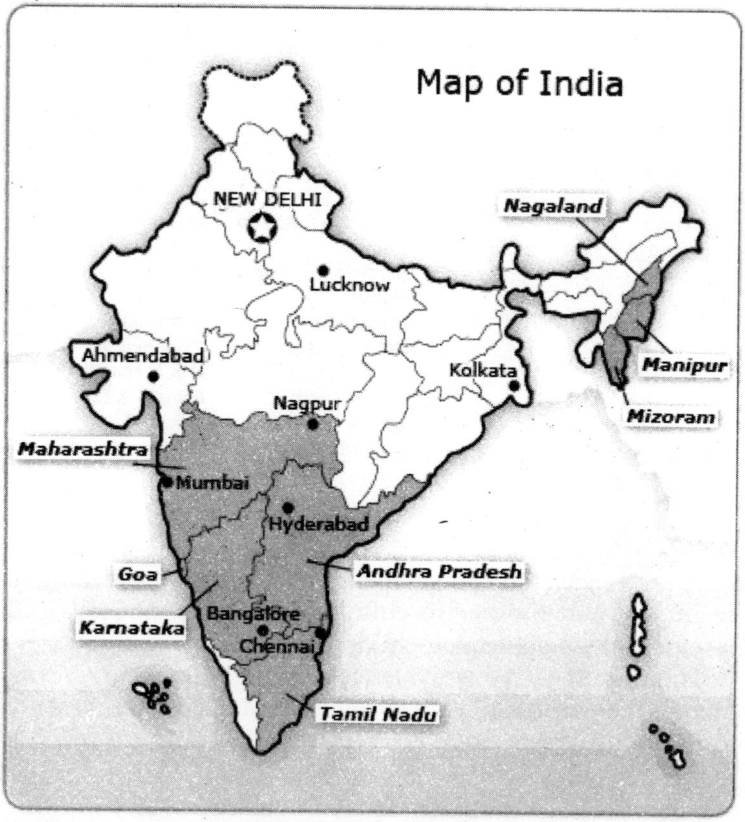

Map 1.2: The Worst Affected States in India

Source: http://www.avert.org/aidsindia.htm

In India, the majority of the HIV/AIDS cases are reported from few states. Although HIV/AIDS still is largely concentrated in at-risk populations, including Commercial Sex Workers (CSWs), Intravenous Drug Users (IDUs), and Men who have Sex with Men (MSM); the surveillance data suggests that the epidemic is moving beyond these groups into the general population; from urban to rural districts; and increasingly towards women and young people (NACO 2006). It is now estimated that many of the HIV cases in India were reported from among housewives with a single partner. The increasing

Table 1.1: Categories of States and Union Territories

High Prevalence	*Moderate Prevalence*	*Low Prevalence*	
		Highly Vulnerable	*Vulnerable*
Tamil Nadu	Gujarat	Assam	Arunachal Pradesh
Andhra Pradesh	Goa	Bihar	Haryana
Maharashtra	Pondicherry	Delhi	J&K
Karnataka		Himachal Pradesh	Meghalaya
Nagaland		Kerala	Mizoram
Manipur		Madhya Pradesh	Sikkim
		Punjab	Tripura
		Rajasthan	A & N Islands
		Uttar Pradesh	Chandigarh
		West Bengal	D & N Haveli
		Chhattisgarh	Daman & Diu
		Orissa	Lakshadweep
		Uttaranchal	

Source: NACO, 2006.

HIV prevalence among even the low-risk women is leading to the increase in mother to child transmission of HIV, and therefore infections among children.

The average HIV prevalence among women attending antenatal clinics in India is 0.48 per cent. Much higher rates are found among people attending STD clinics (3.6%), CSWs (5.1%), IDUs (7.2%) and MSM (7.4%) (*www.avert.org*).

Evolution of Concern for HIV/AIDS in India

The HIV/AIDS epidemic in India is now about 20 years old. However, the incidence of HIV continues to be a cause for concern as the virus continues to spread into new areas as well as into low risk population groups. India has seen a concerted effort to combat the epidemic, from the government, non-government as well as international agencies. India was among the first few countries to start sentinel surveillance and it was initiated under the aegis of ICMR in 1985 (NACO 2007). Surveillance data indicate that risk practices are getting diffused and infection rates are continuing to grow vertically among low risk groups like pregnant mothers. The considerable underreporting of HIV/AIDS cases also hides the fact that management and care of the infected and affected individuals will pose a grave challenge to the resources and capacity of the country.

The virus in India has taken different courses in different states since its first detection and has contributed to the heterogeneity of the epidemic within the country. This heterogeneity has been influenced by varied sexual and injecting behaviour patterns among network population groups such as the CSWs and the IDUs as well as bridge population such as the partner visiting the CSW or the IDU who is married or has a sexual partner thereby linking different networks.

Prevention of mother to child transmission is crucial for primary prevention, treatment and care and support for mothers, their children and families. Inadequate prenatal care services, family planning services, inadequate knowledge of HIV status among pregnant women and stigma and discrimination are obstacles to expanding prevention of mother to child transmission.

The HIV/AIDS epidemic is a serious public health problem. As HIV turns into full blown AIDS there will be a marked increase in the mortality and morbidity rates. Life expectancy will fall as has been witnessed in a number of African countries. Those who are the most infected by the HIV/AIDS are also the most sexually and professionally active groups that falls in the age group of 15-49 years. These people will witness a fall in their productivity rate and income and get trapped in a vicious circle of poverty. Individuals and households will find it difficult to cope with the economic hardships associated with increased treatment cost and reduced income due to illness and loss in productivity. At the micro household level, the financing issues include 3 aspects:

1. The expenses borne by households directly for the illness,
2. The associated coping cost for the family members, and
3. The direct income loss due to illness.

Impact would also be felt severely by the health sector and the government, with government health subsidies rising rapidly as a result of a hastily spreading epidemic (Gupta *et al.* 2003).

State Responses

Genesis and extent of response to the epidemic differed across states and played important roles in shaping the epidemic differently in different states. The Indian Government in an endeavour to curb the spread of the epidemic has responded by setting up the National AIDS Control Organization (NACO) to formulate and implement the National AIDS Control Programme (NACP). It is a centrally sponsored scheme, which comprises of Surveillance, Programme Management, Information, Education and Communication (IEC), Blood Safety, Condom Promotion, Control of STDs and Clinical Management. Initially, NACP was planned for a period of 7 years from 1992 to 1999 which was extended up to 2006. The first phase (1992-1999) of the project was financed by the GOI, contributing $14.1 million and IDA credit of $84 million and a WHO co-financing grant of $1.5 million (Action Aid 2006). In addition USAID and DFID are other two important sources of financing. The overall focus of NACP has been prevention and control and these two components receive the major share of the fund allocated followed by the two components of care and support. Some government and quasi-government organizations have also joined hands with NACO in fighting HIV/AIDS in various capacities and forms. Important among these organizations are Steel Authority of India Limited (SAIL), Indian Railways (IR) and the Defense Ministry. Parliamentarians have also come forward to confront HIV/AIDS and the Parliamentarians Forum for HIV/AIDS was established which organized the first ever National Convention of Elected Representatives on HIV/AIDS in 2003. On December 1, 2003, the then Health Minister announced plans to provide free ARVs to all HIV positive new parents and children under 15 in six states with the highest rates of infection.

The first milestone in the evolution of the concern for HIV/ AIDS was the initiation of sentinel surveillance in 1985. Five years later NACO was formed during 1990-1991. In the following year ICMR established its first AIDS research institute in Pune. NACP is also started in phases in the same year. About 10 years later VCCTC was established in Darjeeling District Hospital. In 2006, PPTCT and two years later ART centre was also started there (Table 1.2).

Table 1.2: Chronology of HIV/AIDS and State Response in India

Year	*State's Response*
1985	Sentinel Surveillance activity in blood donors and STD patients under the aegis of ICMR
1986	First Case of HIV infection found among the CSWs of Chennai National AIDS Committee was formed
1986-1992	Denial of the Threat of HIV
1989	HIV infection reported among the IDUs in Manipur
1990-91	National AIDS Control Organization was established
1990-92	Medium term Plan for prevention and raising awareness
1992	ICMR establishes National AIDS Research Institute in Pune
1992-99	National AIDS Control Programme Phase I is started
1999	HIV testing of all blood bottles becomes mandatory under Supreme Court judgment.
1999-2006	National AIDS Control Programme Phase II
1998-2001	Focus on Targeted Intervention
2000-01	NACO starts feasibility studies for prevention of parent to child transmission of HIV with zidovudine and nevirapine
2002	VCCTC at the Darjeeling District Hospital Established on April 1st
2002	National AIDS Prevention and Control Policy
2002-2003	Tripartite agreement between NACO, ICMR and International AIDS Vaccine Initiative signed to facilitate HIV vaccine development and testing in India
2003	Central Government announces the policy to provide highly active anti-retroviral therapy to those who suffer from AIDS
2005	First AIDS Vaccine trial was initiated
2006	PPTCT started at the Darjeeling District Hospital on March 18th
2007-2012	National AIDS Control Programme Phase III
2008[1]	ART Centre inaugurated at Darjeeling District Hospital on December 1st

Source: NACO, 2006., Kishore, 2005., Panda *et al.* 2002, Godbole & Mehendale. 2005, Field notes.

HIV/AIDS in Darjeeling: Historical Context and the Recent Past

Darjeeling is situated in a geographically strategic location. It shares international borders with Bhutan and Nepal. The borders of Bangladesh and China are also very close. In the year 1835, Darjeeling was ceded to the British East India Company by the Rajah of Sikkim (O'Malley 1989; Pinn 1990). Darjeeling as an urban centre came into existence with the entry of the British in this hill station due to their need for a sanatorium and a summer capital (Lama and Chakraborty 2007). The British developed Darjeeling for reasons of its strategic importance and its potential to become a major trading centre (Palit 2007). However, only with the introduction of tea and cinchona plantation did Darjeeling grow as an urban centre (Pinn 1990). With the plantation of tea and cinchona the population of Darjeeling gradually started to grow from 100 in 1835 to 10,000 in 1859 and a staggering 1,73,342 in the early twentieth century (O'Malley 1989). With the growth of Darjeeling as a summer resort, it soon started to attract the people of the plains with its ample business opportunities. Darjeeling was soon flooded with migrants and business was taken over by the people of the plains. The Biharis and the Marwaris controlled the wholesale and retail business and the Gorkhas who were in majority were left to carry out petty business and manual work. This had a profuse impact on their being socio-economically underdeveloped *vis-à-vis* the business communities (Subba 1992). Darjeeling has today developed into a major tourist hot spot and has been connected with the larger global scenario. This exposure to the outside world has also had its negative fall outs. The youth are indulging in drug abuse and the past years have also witnessed large scale migration among them. Due to the lower socio-economic condition and a growing consumerist culture many are out to earn quick money by any means. Prostitution and drug abuse are on the rise. This situation has made Darjeeling highly vulnerable to HIV/AIDS.

Studying HIV/AIDS in Darjeeling

Darjeeling district has witnessed political unrest for many decades now. Unresolved issues concerning identity, political separation from West Bengal, underdevelopment and lack of willingness on the part of the Central and State Governments to resolve these issues has brought about social and economic crisis in the district and particularly in the hilly regions. The

Darjeeling Gorkha Hill Council (DGHC) was formed in 1988, after a long drawn out struggle for a separate state under the leadership of the Gorkha National Liberation Front (GNLF). However, the autonomous body was not given any real powers for development and employment generation. And there was misappropriation of any funds that came to the Council. This lack of vision and integrity on the part of the local leaderships has plunged the district into deeper crisis. In 2008, the GNLF was unceremoniously overthrown by Gorkha Jan Mukhti Morcha (GJMM), which has again spearheaded the campaign for a separate state. The autonomous Hill Council has no elected leaders and was declared defunct. Recently it is being looked after by the District Magistrate of Jalpaiguri district, with no local political participation. Years of political instability and stepmotherly treatment from the Central and State Governments have had tremendous socio-economic repercussions in the hills of Darjeeling. Infrastructural development remains abysmally low. Health facilities, roads, potable drinking water, educational facilities are acutely inadequate to serve the rapidly growing population.

In the context of HIV/AIDS it is important to note that the only three important hospitals (Victoria, Eden and Planters) were established during the British period. In the past 62 years, the government has not deemed it important to establish any new hospitals there. A few private hospitals have recently come up but they cater to a richer clientele. The sub-divisional hospitals, PHCs and the sub-centre are ill-equipped to handle grave illnesses. During the fieldwork it was seen that among the hospital staff, there was not only a lack of correct awareness about HIV/AIDS, they also lacked empathy towards the positive people. This ill-behaviour may have stemmed from the prejudices arising out of inadequate knowledge about the illness.

As far as education is concerned, barring the schools run by the missionaries, the government run schools lack infrastructure to produce well-groomed students. There are also no good colleges in Darjeeling district so many students go to metros like Delhi, Kolkata, Bangaluru and Mumbai to study. There are no universities in the hilly regions of the district. The only university meant for the district is in Siliguri. The hill students therefore have to go elsewhere for higher studies. Being away from home at such a tender age, away from parental and societal control leads many to indulge in risk behaviours. So apart from those students whose parents can afford to send them outside Darjeeling to study, the rest have to make do with whatever is available. These youth are ill-equipped to compete at various levels. They also do not have any vocational training. This has contributed to higher levels of unemployment. This is leading the youth to frustration which in turn is leading to alcohol consumption and drug addiction. Under the intoxication of drugs and alcohol they are also indulging in risk behaviours. It is seen that even most of the students who have passed out from English medium schools have only managed to get employment in BPOs. BPOs with its glitzy lifestyle, in a metro provide one with anonymity to pursue risk habits.

As far as employment in the hills is concerned apart from the tea gardens which are facing closure due to an ever competitive global market, there are no other industries. The hills of Darjeeling are very fertile and produce a variety of fruits and vegetables and cash crops but it is seen that, the hills, like the colonies during colonial rule only serve to supply raw materials. There are no food processing factories in the hills which could be established if the governments desire.

The unpredictable situation of the tea gardens has exerted pressure on many to migrate in search for better livelihood. Many of these people who are unskilled labourers seek employment in the unorganized sectors and are very susceptible to diverse forms of exploitation. Many women come to the cities to work as domestic help. The nature of their jobs make these people financially insecure and long hours of work make it difficult for them to build social networks. In addition to such a financial position, the lack of social network so far away from home creates loneliness.

The youth who decides to stay at home becomes victims of frustration and depression. With no avenue to vent their anger these youth involve in the abuse of substances. Alcohol consumption and drug abuse among the youth of the hills of Darjeeling is common. At the time of fieldwork there were approximately 1200 youth enrolled at the different Indian Red

Cross Society (IRCS) centres of the hills. In 2002, there were 114 alcohol related deaths in the Eden Hospital alone and in 2003 there were 815 enrolled on account of being alcohol dependent, at Kripa Foundation, a rehabilitation centre for drug and alcohol dependents. This indulgence of the youth is also facilitated by the exposure to the outside world. Both these factors are associated with the spread of HIV/AIDS. The sharing of needles among the IDUs and the engagement of these youth in risk behaviour in the intoxicated state makes them vulnerable to HIV/AIDS. The fact that a large number of PLWHA in Darjeeling are former IDUs supports this fact. The location of the region, which shares international border with Nepal and is in close proximity with the North-East states, which are the recognized routes for drug trafficking, also makes it easy for accessing drugs and this also adds fuel to an already volatile situation.

The exposure to the outside world and the lack of employment opportunities has changed the behaviour pattern of the youth in Darjeeling. The changing value system and the dilution of the traditional lifestyle have removed the taboo against sex. Girls have become more open to sex and the lack of economic pursuits has forced many into prostitution. Sexual practices among the youth are changing at a rapid pace due to various influences on their lifestyle.

The region is also poor in terms of the enormous health infrastructure required for the prevention and control of HIV/AIDS. During the time of conducting the field work there were no ART centres, there was only one VCCTC, which unfortunately was not accessible to the rural populace, there were no CD4 cell counting centres and the health personnel were also ill-trained to provide care and support to the PLWHA. The web of all these complex variables has today made Darjeeling very vulnerable and susceptible to the spread of HIV/AIDS.

Rationale of the Study

The HIV/AIDS epidemic puts the socio-economic, cultural and political condition and the public health crisis of the region into sharp focus. HIV/AIDS highlights the exploitation of women, their low socio-economic status, the trafficking of young girls and it exposes the economic crisis and unemployment that pushes youth into drug addiction and it throws into sharp focus the explosive spread of intravenous drug use in the region (Panos 1999). So in order to implement the desired interventions, the epidemiology of HIV/AIDS in a particular region has to be understood especially with regards to various socio-demographic factors, level of awareness as well as patterns of risk behaviour of the population. The most effective approaches available for the prevention and control of the infection are awareness generation and lifestyle changes.

The area of study has been selected due to the rapid spread of HIV/AIDS in the recent past. Till 2005 about 65 people were detected with the killer disease. The number of cases doubled in the last two years. By November 2007, it had increased to 141. NACO categorizes Darjeeling as a district with increased presence of vulnerable population.

The study region has a large number of drug addicts due to its close proximity to Siliguri and the north-eastern states, which is one of the most important routes for drugs entering into other parts of India from Myanmar. The HIV prevalence among the IDUs was found to be 10-14 per cent in Darjeeling in a survey conducted by the government in 2003-04 which makes the region one with the highest prevalence of HIV among IDUs in the state of West Bengal (IRCS, Kurseong). Siliguri, a commercial centre, is a part of Darjeeling district and also the link between North-East, Sikkim, Bhutan, Nepal and rest of India, not only cater to the drug demands of Darjeeling alone but it also caters to the sexual demands of Darjeeling and its neighbouring places as it has a brothel based sex industry.

All these factors make Darjeeling very prone to HIV/AIDS. It is not just the brothel of Siliguri which acts as a vector for the transmission of the disease to the hills of Darjeeling but also the unorganized sex market available in the hills itself which is posing a great danger for the explosion of HIV/AIDS in the hills.

There is a serious shortage of employment opportunities in the hills of Darjeeling which is forcing the people to migrate.

As a result there is a large influx of people migrating from the hills in search of livelihoods to other parts of India, which also has a great potential for spreading HIV/AIDS in the hills. The political condition of the hills of Darjeeling is also conducive for the spread of HIV/AIDS. Health department comes under the jurisdiction of the DGHC but due to its dissolution, there is no one to take accountability for the intolerable condition of the health sector in the entire hills of Darjeeling. Though the health department is under its jurisdiction, DGHC has not been able to demand for the establishment of an ARV distribution centre in the district hospital. Apart from voluntary counselling and testing the district hospital does not perform any other functions associated with the prevention and control, care and treatment elements of HIV/AIDS.

The political unrest in the hills also favour the spread of HIV/AIDS. With the renewed demand for Gorkhaland strikes and 'bandhs' have become the norm of the day and these are in turn hampering the health seeking behaviour of the PLWHA, as they have to go to North Bengal Medical College and Hospital (NBMCH) at Siliguri, (80-90 kms from Darjeeling) for their check-ups and medicine. The infrastructure of health system is also not developed enough to tackle the rapid growth of HIV/AIDS in the hills of Darjeeling.

The awareness level among the people regarding HIV/AIDS is very low and a lot of misconceptions regarding HIV/AIDS exist among the people. The study area is also part of a district which is considered a high prevalence district in West Bengal. Thus drug addiction, alcoholism, unemployment and political instability is compounding the vulnerability of the area to HIV/AIDS. The area presents a major challenge to public health due to the debilitating effects of HIV/AIDS and the lack of infrastructure to combat the crisis.

Conceptual Framework

HIV/AIDS is rooted in the socio-economic and political conditions of a region and its people. The socio-economic condition of Darjeeling hills is very conducive to the spread of HIV/AIDS. The economy of Darjeeling is to a large extent dependent on tea industries. With the advent of cheaper tea from other parts of the world, the exclusive Darjeeling tea lost a major portion of its market share due to its high price. This has lead to the closure of many tea industries which could not compete in the world market. This had an enormous effect on the economic conditions of the people. Many people lost their livelihood and were rendered homeless and were pushed to poverty. These factors along with sex are recognized factors for HIV/AIDS (Collins and Rau 2000) and the people of Darjeeling hills have been affected by them. Many had to migrate in search of a livelihood. Living far away from home and outside the familiar social network may have forced many of them to engage in risk behaviours. In such a scenario there is a greater chance of them getting infected and transmitting the virus to their spouse at home.

Many young boys of the region join the armed forces. There are probabilities that they indulge in risk behaviour when away from home. Soldiers live far away from their home and families. They are under constant pressure and especially in stressful conditions and environment and are in search for recreation to relieve their stress and loneliness. Peer pressure also leads to risk behaviour and generally the military ethos tends to excuse risky behaviour (McKee *et al.* 2004). Thus, they are likely to be exposed to the HIV infection and in turn render their wives vulnerable to the infection.

The out migration from Darjeeling is largely caused by negligible employment opportunities. One of the recent trends in migration is of women migrating as domestic help, not just to other parts of India but also to foreign countries. This is a major cause of concern as these women do not have any negotiating power and may be exploited sexually which makes them vulnerable to HIV. Lack of employment opportunities can be frustrating and many youths are attracted to drugs and alcohol. Drug addiction and alcoholism, which encourages risk behaviours is very prevalent in the hills. Drug addicts are shunned and looked down upon by the general population so they are confined to their groups and needle sharing among the intravenous drug users is high (Sundas 2004) This practice of needle sharing among them poses greater likelihood of HIV transmission. Female drug addicts, though far less in number than their male counterparts, are more susceptible to being infected by HIV as they face the double danger of being infected through needle sharing as well as sexual intercourse.

Tourism is also an important source of economy in Darjeeling. There is a large influx of tourists every year from around the world. There is a chance that the local population may get infected from the infected tourists in case of contact. There are a large number of sex workers who provide private services. They do not confine their work to Darjeeling town but also travel to nearby places and are likely to have among their clientele the tourists and the nouveau riche especially the contractors. According to a study conducted by NICED, the only brothel in the district is located in Siliguri and it poses immense risk of HIV/AIDS to the hills of Darjeeling as those who cannot afford the services of the Flying Sex Workers (FSWs)[2] in Darjeeling avail the services of these CSWs. The sero-prevalence among the sex workers of this brothel was found to be highest (15.6%) in the whole of West Bengal. To compound the severity of the matter the sex workers also lack awareness and knowledge about methods of prevention of HIV transmission (NICED 2006).

The Voluntary Counselling and Confidential Testing Centre has started in Darjeeling. There is still a shortage of trained personnel. Also one VCCTC in Darjeeling will not suffice for the whole of the hills as it becomes very difficult for those residing in rural areas and in remote areas to access it. Blood safety measures also need upgradation in many of the rural as well as sub-divisional hospitals. As the health delivery systems falls far below the required standard, for the control and prevention of HIV/AIDS, the burden of treatment cost falls directly on the patients and their family. The travel cost is huge as they have to travel to Siliguri or Kolkata for better treatment and care.

The economic burden on those infected and affected by the disease is very huge as the cost of medicine (ARV) is high, beyond the reach of many in the hills and other related expenditures like travel, nutrition etc. also becomes high. The economic burden is much higher when it is compared with the economic conditions of those who are not affected, as the per capita income of the people in these areas is low. People in search of treatment will be in the danger of losing their life long savings and other assets but all will be in vain as there is no therapeutic treatment for HIV/AIDS till date.

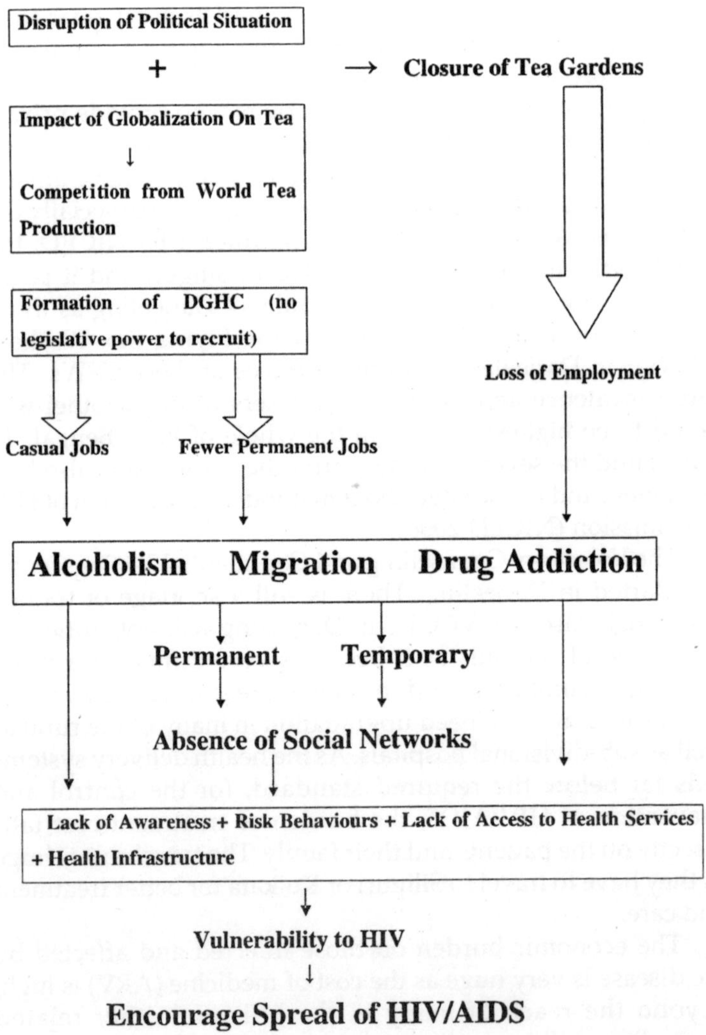

Fig. 1.1: Conceptual Framework of Factors Associated with HIV/AIDS in Darjeeling Hills

Analytical Framework

The analytical framework of the present study includes a discussion on research question and purpose of the study followed by the hypothesis and the research design.

Research Questions

The political situation of Darjeeling is volatile. The socio-economic conditions are rapidly changing. There is growing trend towards westernization. The above factors along with the present day dismal infrastructure of health system, educations etc. have grave implications on the health of the people. The dangers of HIV/AIDS are more pronounced in such situation. The following research questions are designed to arrive at a clear picture of the presence and threat of HIV/AIDS in the study area:

(1) What are the main determinants of the spread of HIV/AIDS in Darjeeling hills?
(2) Which sections of the society have been affected by HIV/AIDS?
(3) What is the level of awareness of HIV/AIDS among the people and what programmes are implemented to raise awareness?
(4) How do the community members perceive HIV/AIDS?
(5) What are the important consequences of HIV/AIDS on the families of those infected?
(6) What is the available infrastructure in terms of health clinics, treatment, care and counselling and testing centres?
(7) What has been the state and institutional responses to confront the disease?

Objectives

Thus the main objectives of the study are—

- To study the provision, planning and management of HIV/AIDS services.

- To look at the implications of migration on the spread of HIV/AIDS in Darjeeling.
- To look at how the administrative structure of the region is responsible for the strategies and plans to address HIV/AIDS
  - What is the role of DGAHC?
  - What is the role of major employers such as the tea gardens and railways?
  - What is the role of other agencies (which are working and funding for the control and prevention of HIV/AIDS in the region)?
  - What is the level of success of the current modes of HIV/AIDS prevention and control adopted by the state and other concerned institutions?

Hypothesis

The poor socio-economic conditions of the people of Darjeeling hills since independence and the lack of infrastructure in terms of quality education, health facilities, employment avenues etc. has had an adverse effect on the society. This has pushed people towards risk behaviour, making the environment conducive to HIV/AIDS.

Research Design

Study Area

The study comprises of the three hill sub-divisions of Darjeeling district—Darjeeling, Kalimpong and Kurseong, which are situated in the northern part of the state of West Bengal. The study area was selected because it is part of Darjeeling district which has a high HIV prevalence among the IDUs and also among the women visiting antenatal care. The study area is labelled as Darjeeling hills for the purpose of the study.

Methodology

The present study incorporates review of literature and published data; and a field based data collection and analysis.

Literature on the global and Asian scenario of HIV/AIDS as well as that of India has been extensively reviewed. Relevant data from sources such as UNAIDS, UNDP, NACO and WBSAP&CS have been analyzed.

As part of the field study, data have been collected by employing qualitative as well as quantitative methods from the sample derived using purposive sampling and snowball techniques. The respondents comprises of community members, PLWHA, flying sex workers[3], intravenous drug users and bisexuals.[4] The purposive sampling was used to identify the respondents from among the community members while snowball technique was used to draw sample from among FSWs, IDUs, PLWHA and bisexuals.

The methodology also included a case study of Shanker Foundation and other NGOs from the Darjeeling hills who were involved in the control and prevention of HIV/AIDS. NGOs were also visited for the conduct of in-depth interviews and observations of the implementation of the programmes. Participation in the programmes of the NGOs was also done to get a first hand knowledge of the way these NGOs functioned.

The data collection was undertaken from the month of July to December in 2007. Prior to the data collection, preliminary work was conducted on two field visits to the study area to establish relations with the key informants and the PLWHA. Before going to the field for data collection literature review was also done.

Tools and Techniques

Multiple methods were used for data collection, including non-participatory observation among the PLWHA and IDUs, in-depth interviews, informal conversations and focus group discussions.

Focus group discussion was also carried out among three groups. One group was those of FSWs and the other group was of the community members and the third group was of the IDUs. Unfortunately not many came for the discussion and there were no female participants among the community members and the IDUs. There were only 4 participants in the focus group discussion conducted among the community members, 5 among the FSWs and 7 among the IDUs (Tables 1.3, 1.4 and 1.5). The focus group discussion for the community members was conducted in Kurseong, with the IDUs it was conducted in Darjeeling and with the FSWs it was also conducted in Kalimpong. The participants were educated, married, single and divorced. Still it provided an in-depth knowledge of important issues from the perspective of the participants. Guidelines for the discussion were prepared and used for the same to seek spontaneous responses from the participants.

Table 1.3: Characteristics of the Participants in the Focus Group Discussion (FSW)

Sl. No	*Age*	*Sex*	*Marital Status*	*Education*	*Income*
1	30	F	Married	12th	2500
2	26	F	Married	7th	3500
3	23	F	Single	12th	5000-6000
4	29	F	Single	12th	6000
5	25	F	Married	10th	5000

Source: Field Data.

Table 1.4: Characteristics of the Participants in the Focus Group Discussion (Community Members)

Sl. No	*Age*	*Sex*	*Marital Status*	*Education*	*Income*
1	25	M	Single	B.A.	3500
2	32	M	Married	B.A.	12,000
3	25	M	Single	12th	2000
4	24	M	Single	12th	Nil

Source: Field Data.

Field notes were the salient method of data recording. Five groups of respondents formed the study population, the community members (public), 'the flying sex workers (FSWs),' the IDUs, PLWHA and the bisexuals. A semi-structured interview schedule was designed to collect primary data while a desk survey of relevant literature and organizational documents was done to collect secondary data.

Table 1.5: Characteristics of the Participants in the Focus Group Discussion (IDUs)

Sl. No	Age	Sex	Marital Status	Education	Income
1	27	M	Single	B.A.	Nil
2	30	M	Married	B.A.	8000
3	29	M	Single	B.A.	Nil
4	25	M	Single	12th	2000
5	33	M	Divorced	M.A.	9000
6	32	M	Married	7th	3000
7	26	M	Married	B.A.	8000

Source: Field Data.

A number of in-depth interviews were also carried out to acquire greater knowledge on the prevalence of HIV/AIDS, awareness and perception of the community members about HIV/AIDS, and stigma and discrimination faced by those infected and affected by the disease. Some data was collected through case studies done in all the 3 sub-divisions. Knowledgeable persons working in the area of HIV/AIDS were also interviewed as key informants and utmost care was taken to involve diverse sections of the society.

Choice of Language

The choice of language was Nepali and English. Nepali was chosen, as this is the *lingua franca* of the region, so it made the communication with the respondents easier. Speaking in the local language also helped to establish a cordial relationship thereby making the interview process easier. The choice of language was left to the respondents. English was also chosen as many were conversant in it.

The Interview Process

In order to ensure confidentiality and emphasize the voluntary nature of the interview all potential respondents were asked for prior appointments to ensure their convenience and were also given the choice of opting out of the interview. Moreover, even on the day of contact the researcher ensured that respondents could opt out, or negotiate a better time and place for the interview. The purpose of the interview was always explained and interviews lasted for 30-120 minutes.

Semi-structured schedule was used for interviewing. Most of the interviews were carried out in Nepali and only 10 interviews were carried out in English. It was designed to elicit spontaneous replies to open ended questions. The interview covered the subject's views on how HIV/AIDS is transmitted, what are the ways to prevent it, who are the most vulnerable population, if they would like to talk, sit and communicate with the PLWHA. The interview also sought to find out the respondents' view on the medical facilities for the welfare and treatment of those who were infected by the disease, and whether or not the PLWHA had to face any problems in accessing these facilities, if available. Importantly, from the key informants information on the political will to control the epidemic was sought.

The PLWHA were selected from Shanker Foundation, Darjeeling. As Shanker Foundation is the only network of positive people of the hill sub-divisions of Darjeeling the researcher was able to interact with PLWHA from different social settings and to generate diverse information on the experiences of the PLWHA. The location of the interview for the PLWHA was the Shanker Foundation office as this was the most convenient place for them to be interviewed without any disturbance and interruption. They were encouraged to seek clarification before the interview began and were also given the option to withdraw from the interview at any point of time. With their permission the interviews were noted down in details by the researcher. Depending on the context of the interview specific phrasing of the questions varied slightly across participants and some other open-ended questions were also asked during the interview process.

Choice of Shanker Foundation

Shanker Foundation was selected as it was the only place where the possibility of meeting all the PLWHA was overwhelmingly positive. Moreover, most of the PLWHA had not disclosed their positive status at the time of interview so there was a chance of at least interviewing those who had disclosed their sero status. All the PLWHA were not known to me except two with whom rapport was developed in the previous visit to Shanker Foundation. It was thought that to develop a good rapport it would be better to meet them in a place where they would be among the people they trusted. Shanker Foundation also helped me to meet all the PLWHA and approach them for interview and in case any one of them declined to be interviewed I had other interviewees.

The first PLWHA agreed to be interviewed only after I had made numerous forays at Shanker Foundation office at Darjeeling. Before the respondent agreed I had to talk with the members of the foundation and convince them that the purpose of the study was academic and was not for any profit making purpose. The members also tested my knowledge of HIV/AIDS and asked questions on discrimination and other aspects of the disease. The most important incident occurred when I had gone there the second day. The coordinator offered me tea and said that people think that the disease can also spread by having tea or for that matter from utensils used by people infected by the virus. To gain their confidence I had to narrate stories of meeting people infected with the virus from India and abroad. After hearing their stories about discrimination I also had to tell them about their rights and also how it was inhuman to discriminate only because somebody was infected by some virus. During this period I had to make sure that I did not hurt their sentiments in any way. After the co-ordinator of the foundation was satisfied, he allowed me to interview his colleagues. The first interview was of a female respondent and she was very honest. At the end of the interview she said that she felt very good talking to me as she could tell me everything she had inside her and so much wanted to share with somebody.

Among the community members almost everybody I interviewed suspected me of something or the other. The first interview I conducted was possible after many rejected the proposal. Many among the community members also inquired whether I was infected or not.

Challenges of the Study

The study is subject to several important challenges. The findings reflect the behaviours and beliefs of a relatively small sample from one specific geographic area. The sample is small because many in the area refused to be interviewed and also many interviews could not be included here as there were inconsistencies and contradictions in the respondents' responses to the questions. Our understanding of knowledge and perception of HIV/AIDS are inferred from retrospective reports, rather than measured over time. More importantly, the large imbalance in the ratio between male and female respondents raises the possibility of selective bias for the male sample.

Some respondents were skeptical and suspicious regarding the motive and attitude of the researcher. Due to this reason many whom the researcher wanted to interview did not oblige. Many were too hesitant to talk about issues like sex, sexual behaviour and HIV/AIDS. The views of many people involved in the field of HIV/AIDS, like the secretary of DACC, the CMO of Kurseong Sub-Divisional Hospital could not be sought because of their time constraints and also as many did not want to give any interview. Only a few politicians were interviewed as they were either not available or denied talking about HIV/AIDS saying that it was not their concern and it came under the purview of the health department.

Only 11 PLWHA were interviewed as many had not disclosed their status and their identity was not known. Except one who was interviewed at Kalimpong, only those coming to Shanker Foundation and willing to give interview were interviewed. Out of the five PLWHA who had disclosed their status only two could be interviewed as one of them was in a rehabilitation centre in Sikkim and the other two were out of station, attending training programmes and official work of Shanker Foundation. The number of care givers is less in the sample as many of the PLWHA had not even disclosed their HIV sero positive status to their family. Due to some problem in bureaucratic protocol the report taken out by DACC for the area it covers was also not made available to the researcher. The interviews were desired to be one to one but some of the interviews had to be executed in the presence of someone or the other. Subjects may have underreported the number of persons with whom they had injected or had had sex with as they did not want to mention knowing certain other drug injectors or sex partners. Since the subjects were recruited through purposive and snowballing sampling technique the data may also have limited representation. In spite of these challenges, the data has provided the opportunity to make a number of important inferences. It must also be borne in mind that the data are derived from self-report. Furthermore, all information is largely retrospective.

HIV/AIDS: Review of Literature

Under the aegis of ICMR in 1985, India was among the first few countries to initiate sentinel surveillance (NACO 2007). The impact of HIV/AIDS will be felt severely by the health sector and the government, with government health subsidies rising rapidly as a result of a hastily spreading epidemic the government will also feel the burden of the epidemic as it will have to subsidise health care immensely (Gupta *et al.* 2003). As per the UNAIDS report 2007 there are 2.31 million people currently infected by HIV. NACO Annual Report (2004) gives a comprehensive picture of the epidemic in India. It divides the states of India into high, moderate and low prevalence states and brings out a clear scenario of the disease in each of these states.

The report finds that:

1. AIDS is increasingly affecting young people in the sexually active age group. The majority of the HIV infections (87.7%) are in the age group of 15-44 years.
2. The predominant mode of transmission of the HIV infection is through heterosexual contact (85.7%), followed by injecting drug use (2.2%), blood transfusion and blood product infusion (2.6%), perinatal transmission as 2.7 per cent and others as 6.8 per cent.
3. In the HIV sentinel surveillance 2003, males accounted for 73.5 per cent of AIDS cases and females 26.5 per cent. The ratio between male and female was approximately 3:1.

4. The predominant opportunistic infection among AIDS patients is tuberculosis, indicating a potential future spread of the HIV-TB co-infection.

There is an absence of vaccine or drug to cure the disease (Kalichman 1998) and this has led to further spread of the epidemic. Although HIV/AIDS is concentrated among the high risk groups there are evidences that it is moving beyond them and into the low risk population like the women and youth (NACO 2006).

The search for vaccines that could potentially impede the relentless increase in the number of the people infected by HIV cannot be accomplished without the involvement of large pharmaceutical companies. But these companies have hardly shown any interest in searching and producing AIDS vaccines as the countries severely suffering from the AIDS epidemic cannot afford to buy these vaccines in quantities enough for them to achieve minimum profit (Craddock 2007).

Determinants of HIV/AIDS

Poverty, sex work and migration are acknowledged socio-economic risk factors for HIV (Collins and Rau 2000). Poverty encourages the spread of HIV and quicker progression from HIV sero-positivity to full blown AIDS (Masanjala 2007). Poverty and inequality can drive those on the margin of destitution into risky livelihood and coping strategies that raise their likelihood of contracting HIV. AIDS overwhelmingly affects individuals living in underdeveloped countries, where poverty and lack of access to resources such as health care, ARVs continues to drive the epidemic. Although AIDS is not simply diseases of the poor, determinants of the epidemic go far beyond individual volition and that some dimensions of being poor increases risk and vulnerability to HIV (Dodoo *et al.* 2007; Masanjala 2007). Economic hardship is acknowledged to compound women's sexual vulnerability. Economic stresses associated with low wages, unemployment and poverty leads many women to use sex to generate income for basic needs provoking early initiation of sexual activity and high incidence of multiple sexual partners (Ulin 1992). These conditions also promote men to exploit women's economic vulnerability by paying very little for sex and subjecting women to domestic violence (Dodoo *et al.* 2007). Dodoo *et al.* further examines the relationship between economic circumstances and sexual outcomes across urban and rural Kenya. Although poverty is significantly associated with the sexual outcomes in all settings the urban poor are significantly more likely than their rural counterparts to have an early sexual debut and a greater incidence of multiple sexual partners. They compare the impact of socio-economic deprivation on risky sexual outcomes in rural and urban Kenya. The disadvantage of the urban poor is accentuated for married women and those in Nairobi's slums are at least three times as likely to have multiple partners as their rural counterparts. The determinants to vulnerability should be recognized as rooted in poverty, social disruption, underemployment, gender and access to resources (Social Science & Medicine 2007). For women vulnerabilities to HIV are exacerbated by widespread gender based social inequalities (Oppong 1998). HIV/AIDS highlights the exploitation encountered by women which is a fallout of their low socio-economic status (Panos 1999). Yet the dominant biomedical paradigm of AIDS research continues to centre upon individual behaviour rather than looking at the social and economic contexts (MacDonald 1996).

Condom has become an effective barrier against HIV/AIDS. However, its use is not very widespread among the people. Significant proportion of young people experience risky or unwanted sexual activity within the context of marriage and in premarital relationships and they do not receive prompt or appropriate care and experience adverse reproductive health outcomes including HIV/AIDS (Santhya *et al.* 2007). Married women constitute a group with distinct risk of HIV/AIDS and face a host of obstacles in making informed decisions in protecting themselves from infections. Findings from a number of studies conducted among HIV positive women also show that a substantial proportion of infected women were young women whose only HIV risk factor was sex with their spouse (NACO 2006). In societies where there is a prevalence of multiple sexual partners, where prostitution is a major component of sexual culture and where premarital sex is universal there is a likelihood of very rapid transmission of HIV/AIDS (Ford and Koetsawang 1991). Despite the increasing information on the risk of sexual relations without the protection of a condom people continue to be involved in this risk behaviour (Munoz-Silva *et al.* 2007).

Stigma and Discrimination

Wiess & Ramakrishna (2006) defines stigma as "a social process or related personal experience characterized by exclusion, rejection, blame or devaluation that results from experience of reasonable anticipation of an adverse social judgment about a person or group identified with a particular health problem." Link and Phelan (2006) conceptualize stigma as a process in which five interrelated components are connected to lead to stigma. They are "labelling, stereotyping separation between people who label and the labelled, experience of discrimination and loss of status in the labelled and finally the exercise of power by those who do the labelling and stereotyping, which translates negativity and undesirability for the labelled." Ever since the epidemic began PLWHA have been victims of stigmatization. The degree of stigma and discrimination associated with AIDS is the greatest compared to other infections (Crawford 1996). Discrimination related with HIV/AIDS is also compounded by the public's negative attitude towards high risk groups such as CSWs (Peracca *et al.* 1998). General ignorance and misconceptions about HIV/AIDS have been the primary reasons for this discrimination (Zhou 2007). The negative responses and attitude towards PLWHA are related to the general levels of knowledge about HIV/AIDS and in particular to the causes of AIDS and the routes of HIV transmission (Bharat 2001). Within an environment where PLWHA are stigmatized and shunned, they conceal their status and if they do not disclose their sero status to their partners, friends and family they will not receive desirable help, care and support. Discrimination occurs when a person is treated unfairly and unjustly because he or she is perceived to be deviant from others or to belong to a particular group. Discrimination manifests in three major forms—overt, subtle and insidious, whereby stigmatized individuals realize that they have been labelled and have consequently lost their social status and also that stigma has both direct and indirect import on health (Link and Phelan 2006). The consequences of insidious discriminations include strained interactions, more restricted social networks and support, unemployment and loss of income (Deng *et al.* 2007). However, stigma and discrimination associated with HIV/AIDS stems from the underlying stigmatization of sex and intravenous drug use, both being the main paths of HIV transmission (UNAIDS 2003). There is a widespread discrimination towards PLWHA everywhere. Despite their knowledge and understanding about HIV/AIDS the perception of the PLWHA about and the response to HIV/AIDS is to a large extent influenced by their experiences of interactions with the others. The major implication of stigma and discrimination is that it creates a vicious cycle of social isolation, marginalization and thus addiction relapse (Deng *et al.* 2007). The prevention of HIV/AIDS should not be limited to the awareness of the infection but it should also focus on discrimination and stigma (Zhou 2007). Li *et al.* (2007) says that the Chinese professionals display more judgmental attitudes and less willingness to interact even casually with hypothetical patient with HIV/AIDS than with Hepatitis B. They further say that higher status medical professionals with more medical education and those occupying positions with more medical facilities showed more prejudice attitude towards PLWHA and less willingness to have social interaction with AIDS patients. Medical education in general and education about HIV/AIDS in particular will not necessary reduce the stigma and discrimination attached with HIV/AIDS unless it reduces specific fears of infection in the workplace. This has to be coupled with access to necessary equipment and procedures to ensure that health professionals can manage the risk of workplace infection appropriately (Deacon and Boulle 2007).

A study, 'AIDS Discrimination in Asia' (2004) conducted by the Positive People's Network of India with the support of ILO, found that about 92 per cent of the respondents were in the age-group 19-40 years, the most productive age-group. This study also shows that expenditure on medicines and food increased as a result of an infected person in the family, and, expenditure on education and entertainment decreased, which had an adverse impact on the quality of life of all the family members. Children were losing their parents due to AIDS which in turn put the responsibility of these children on the old grandparents who themselves were in need of support. This report documents a peer-led study on AIDS-related stigma and discrimination of people living with HIV and AIDS (PLWHA) in Asia. Findings show that over 80 per cent of respondents experienced some form of discrimination in the health sector, the community, the family and the workplace. Other findings included: lack of pre-test counselling, forced testing, treatment refusal and breaches of confidentiality. The report also highlights how women are significantly more likely than men to experience discrimination within the family and the community.

In India, as elsewhere, AIDS is perceived as a disease of 'others'—of people living on the margins of society, whose lifestyles are considered perverted and deviant. Discrimination, stigmatization, and denial are the expected outcomes of such values, affecting life in families, communities, workplaces, schools, and health care settings (Bharat 2001). There exists no research in Darjeeling dealing with how PLWHA or those suspected of being HIV sero positive are perceived and treated because of their illness. However, it is quite evident from studies done in other parts of the globe that the PLWHA are not fairly treated and discriminated against because of their HIV/AIDS status (Aggleton 2000). PLWHA are stigmatized and discriminated against because their illness is primarily perceived to be contagious and threatening and not understood fully by the lay people. HIV/AIDS stigma and discrimination interfere with HIV/AIDS prevention, diagnosis and treatment and can become internalized by PLWHA (Simbayi *et al.* 2007). In India it is the women who are treated improperly than the men when found to be HIV positive. The women have to go through all the ordeals and are chased away from home, are not given the ancestral property (Bharat 2001). Stigma and discrimination may cause PLWHA to face social isolation, increased emotional distress and a loss of socio-economic support (FHI 2004). The PLWHA in the hills of Darjeeling are a hidden population as HIV/AIDS is the most 'stigmatized medical condition in the world' (Simbayi 2007; Kalichman 2007). The health officials in many parts of India are not well aware and well informed about HIV/AIDS and its treatment, especially those in the lower rungs of the hierarchy (*www.avert.org*), The growth rate has brought into action a variety of actors for its control and prevention. A variety of interventions have been implemented targeting diverse population. There has also been a wide spectrum of responses at the international, national and the local level. Yet the Indian public has not been well informed and active participants to confront the challenges posed by HIV/AIDS as there are very few sources of cogent information available about HIV/AIDS that people have access to (Ramasubban and Rashyasringa ed. 2005). 'The Medecins Sans Frontiers' expressed concern that access to affordable medicines for HIV/AIDS was becoming bleak (*www.accessmed-msf.org* 2005). In July 2005, the leaders of the G8 countries at the Gleneagles Summit committed to 'developing and implementing a package for HIV prevention, treatment and care with the aim of coming as close as possible to the goal of universal access to treatment by 2010 for all those who need it' (UNAIDS 2006).

A Report by the Positive People's Network of India (2004), states that serious and harmful discrimination against PLWHA prevails even in countries with progressive anti-discrimination legislation. Protecting the rights of PLWHA enables individual members of society to examine their vulnerability to HIV infection and that this is the most effective way to improve public health outcomes for all people.

Migration and HIV/AIDS

The fear that people coming from other countries and regions might bring dangerous contagious diseases into societies is deeply rooted among the people, ever since the Black Death (Knipe and Rector 2002). The epidemic seems to be more significant among the lower socio-economic groups mostly being migrants (Annual Report, WBSAP&CS, 2005-06). Mostly it is the young, often at the peak of their reproductive and sexual productivity, who are most readily displaced because of economic deprivation and the lure of the city. Their uprooting and movement to urban centres or other countries can involve a dramatic divorce from traditional values and the social control which the family and the society structure exercise over their sexual behaviour (Carballo and Siem 2002). Migration in search of livelihood is conducive to the spread of HIV/AIDS as it places men and women in particular risk situation, in which institutions providing normal social support for stable family relations are absent (Collins and Rau 2001). Among the migrants, peer influences on risk behaviour have been documented among a number of groups (Imem and Suwannarat 2002).

The UNDP's report on HIV and Migration (2004) examines the factors pertaining to HIV and migration in countries of South and North-East Asia. It highlights the increasing level of mobility and the context and conditions in which it occurs, which in turn affects the vulnerability of the migrants and their families to HIV. The report says that although all the seven countries have started to acknowledge that the HIV/AIDS epidemic poses a serious challenge, there are huge differences in the extent of commitment of each country and the resources available to tackle the epidemic. Further the absence of studies, data and information that explore issues concerning vulnerabilities of specific sub-groups within migrant workers has contributed further to the lack of comprehensive responses directed at migrant workers and their communities. The inter-country migrants are more vulnerable than in-country migrants because of a host of reasons. Their vulnerability stems from language barriers feeling of alienation, distance and long periods of absence from home, limited access to information and services, limited rights to organize and negotiate for better services and fear of deportation upon testing positive for HIV. The report says that countries like Bangladesh and Sri Lanka provide pre-departure training for outgoing migrants. However, these training either do not address HIV/AIDS or do so only minimally. The study found that there are very small number of models of good practice—where they do exists, they are limited in their scope and impact. The report says that unless Asian governments and international organizations respond quickly, the effect of the epidemic in the region could be devastating.

Human mobility is an overriding factor responsible for the spread of infectious diseases, particularly at the start of newly emerging or reemerging epidemics such as HIV/AIDS and

SARS (Komatsu and Sawada 2007). The emergence of previously unknown infectious diseases, such as AIDS combined with the increased speed and volume of international trade and travel, have made countries conscious of their vulnerability to new and emerging infectious disease threats that can easily cross borders (Fidler 2004). All countries are vulnerable to the outbreaks either they emerge within national borders or present threats through international spread or decreased investment in public health has increased such vulnerability.

As the employment opportunities in the hills of Darjeeling are few there are many people migrating to other parts of the country as well to foreign countries in search of employment. Migration in search of livelihood is conducive to the spread of HIV/AIDS as it places men and women in particular risk situation, in which institutions providing normal social support for stable family relations are absent (Collins and Rau 2001). Migrants are more likely to be in high-risk situations since they are often poor, live away from their families and are more likely to engage in unprotected sex. Indeed, while there is no systematic information on this subject, government surveys indicate that most people who learn of their HIV status can trace their infection to a sexual encounter outside the state (Srinivasan and Sukumar 2006).

Intravenous Drug Users and HIV/AIDS

The association between injecting drugs and HIV transmission has been well established. However, this risk behaviour persists in most of the countries in the world and HIV infection associated with injecting drug in many of these countries has been found. The epidemic is sustained at high levels due to the dynamic interaction between high risk needle and syringe sharing, the high prevalence rate which increases the odds of sharing injecting equipment with an HIV positive partner, the high infectivity of new cases of infection and the extensive mobility and mixing between IDUs (Stimson 2005). Among the intravenous drug users, HIV infection is transmitted primarily through contaminated injection equipment, specifically needles and syringes. Drug paraphernalia is frequently shared by one or more individuals at the time drugs are injected. HIV infected IDUs can also transmit the virus to their sexual partners and wives, who may or may not themselves be IDUs (Rhodes and Malotte 1996).

Asia has seen the most rapid diffusion of HIV infection among IDUs. In Manipur the first HIV sero positive IDU was not detected until October 1989, within three months 9 per cent of the IDUs were found to be HIV sero positive, and in the next three months, the prevalence rate had increased to 56 per cent (Sarkar *et al.* 1994; Naik *et al.* 1991). By 1990 it was estimated that there were approximately 15,000 IDUs in Manipur and most were under the age of 25 and needle sharing was common among them (Sarkar *et al.* 1991). Due to this phenomenon high rate of HIV prevalence among the IDUs is found throughout the world. Extremè high prevalence was found among the IDUs of Ruili, China, at 82 per cent in 1992, in Chiang Rai, Thailand it was 61 per cent in 1989, in Myanmar rates of above 60 per cent have been reported from most of the testing sites since sentinel surveillance programme was introduced there in 1992 (Stimson 2005). Majority of the IDUs are males. Most are sexually active with there spouses, casual partners and with female commercial sex workers. Condom use among them is rare. There are evidences of rapid transmission of HIV to the spouses of IDUs sexually. In Manipur within one year of HIV spread among IDUs, 6 per cent of the wives who were tested were found to be HIV positive (*Ibid*). The consistent use of condom among IDUs varies by the subject's HIV sero status and by whether or not the partner in relationship is an IDU. Consequently, the individual may have consistent condom use with one partner but not with another (Freidman *et al.* 2005).

IDUs are also initiated into drug use under peer pressure and influence. It is this social aspect of injecting drugs which involves the sharing of needles and syringes that has given rise to the rapid increasè in the rate of HIV transmission (Ford and Koetsawang 1991).

Women and HIV/AIDS

Women are found to be vulnerable to the onslaught of HIV/AIDS for a host of reasons. The salient reasons seem to the patriarchal nature of the society which restricts women from being aware or negotiate methods of safe sex. There are numerous obstacles posed by culture and traditions in the path of women to be self-reliant on issues of sex and sex education. Their initiatives to learn about safe sex are termed as unwanted and deviant and are socially ostracized if they intend to do that. Consequently, globally the number of women being infected by HIV is increasing. Women are thought to learn about sex after marriage and are thereby exposed to the dangers of being infected by their husbands after marriage. Even the sexual and reproductive health initiatives have focused only on the unmarried young couples assuming that the married couples practice safe sex and do not face any stigma that their unmarried counterparts experience in accessing sexual and reproductive health services. However, emerging evidences suggest that neither of these assumptions is tenable. They are of the opinion that the young married women are at a risk of HIV and face a host of obstacles in making informed sexual and reproductive health decisions (Santhya and Jejebhoy 2007) while leaving the married women who have neither the negotiating power nor the skill to safeguard their sexual health and are exploited within the institution of marriage. Early marriage also enhances young women's HIV risk, however, presumably because married women have less negotiating power and more sexual exposure. They also experience pressure to bear a child, which increase the risk of unprotected sexual intercourse (Clarke 2004). The husband's irresponsible behaviour is also responsible for the exposure of the women to sexual risks. They indulge in extra- marital sex which devoids the wife of sexual pleasure, emotional support from the husband and the economic security which a women looks for in marriage. Under such circumstances many women take to commercial sex to look for the economic security and at times for the emotional support. Some women have reported having multiple partners for attractive consumer goods and to revenge their husband's infidelity (Tawfik and Watkins 2007). Migration of the husbands has also contributed to the risks of women. When women are left behind by the migrating husbands many a times the wives have to find their own means of survival and also provide for their children. Sex work has become a very common option and one of the few sources of employment left open to them (Carbolla and Siem 2002).

Sexual Behaviour and HIV/AIDS

Till date, most of the studies of young people's HIV-related risk behaviours have focused on levels and determinants of condom use and sexual activity (Eaton *et al.* 2003) or on the social aspects of HIV/AIDS risk, such as unequal gender and power relations and sexual coercion (Wood *et al.* 1998). The advent of HIV/AIDS in the world has brought attention to sexual behaviour and partnership. Sexual relationships with multiple partners are associated with an increased risk of acquiring HIV/AIDS infection (Gregson *et al.* 2002). However, economic hardship may also motivate young women to employ their sexual resources to meet their economic demands.

Unequal power between the sexual partners often plays out in the arena of reproductive decision-making, causing women to be unable to control the timing of sex or to initiate safe sexual behaviour (Ankrah 1991). A woman's inability to refuse sex is closely related to her inability to avoid becoming infected with HIV/AIDS. A woman can refuse sex to multiple partners and can be monogamous. However, in the context of marriage she is over-powered by the desires and the wishes of her husband. Therefore, she cannot initiate safe sex or the timings of sex.

It needs to be borne in mind that the reporting of sexual behaviour is widely recognized to incorporate biases (Gregson *et al.* 2002) and are often rooted in gender considerations. Men are more likely to exaggerate the number of sexual partners and women are likely to underreport the number of sexual partners. Premarital sex is considered to be associated with risky behaviour which may result in increased prevalence of HIV/AIDS. The weakening of family and social control and the changing social, political and economic environment also has an impact on the sexual behaviour of the young people. The earlier the sexual debut of the young people there are more chances that they will indulge in risk behaviour and infection of HIV/AIDS. Men who are involved in substance abuse frequently indulge in risk behaviour.

The themes of study for understanding the dynamics of HIV/AIDS in different parts of the world are as diverse as the strains of HIV. The reasons for the dissemination of HIV/AIDS are also diverse. Taking this into consideration a lot of studies have been done using a perspective that would help to understand in greater details, the reasons for the spread of HIV/AIDS, the variables associated with it, the policy that need to be implemented for the control and prevention of it. However, not many studies have been done in the region of Darjeeling hills.[5] The reasons for the spread of HIV/AIDS in the hills of Darjeeling are similar and pertinent as in other parts of the world. Unfortunately, till recent times the control and prevention of HIV/AIDS was neglected by the government in the hills of Darjeeling. This research is an endeavour to understand the dynamics of HIV/AIDS, the responses to control and prevent it, the care and support the PLWHA are receiving from different agencies and the understanding of HIV/AIDS epidemic by the community and society at large.

Design of the Study

The introductory chapter is designed to profile an overview of the crisis of HIV/AIDS in the world and also the responses it has elicited. It further discusses the methodology; tools and techniques of data collection; the reasons for selecting the study area and the problems faced in conducting the research. The second section of the chapter is the review of literature on HIV/AIDS and brings out the different themes depicted in the large corpus of literature associated with the study of HIV/AIDS.

The second chapter gives a brief socio-political history of Darjeeling and also discusses the risk factors associated with HIV/AIDS and prevalence in the study area. It discusses the advent of HIV/AIDS in Darjeeling and highlights the profile of Shanker Foundation—a network of positive people in Darjeeling.

The third chapter titled 'Socio-Demographic Profile of the Study Population' deals with the socio-demographic conditions of the sample population and also analyses in detail each category of the groups of people that make up the sample population. The chapter profiles the PLWHA and highlights their various experiences.

The fourth chapter deals with mobility, sexual behaviour

and trends among the people, risk groups, the knowledge and perception of HIV/AIDS among the people and also the stigma and discrimination associated with HIV/AIDS in the hills of Darjeeling.

The fifth chapter gives a brief account of international response to HIV/AIDS and primarily focuses on the responses from various institutions in the hills of Darjeeling, to control and prevent the epidemic.

The sixth chapter discusses the spread of HIV/AIDS through population mobility, use of technology, substance abuse, sexual behaviour, knowledge and experiences of the infected and affected persons. The chapter also illustrates the findings and proposes some strategies to address the epidemic in Darjeeling hills. The concluding chapter deals with the summary of the study and based on these draws conclusions.

Notes and References

1. This ART Centre came into existence after the field-work was carried out.
2. They are called flying sex workers as they are not confined to any place and can carry out their business anywhere.
3. The sex workers in Darjeeling are called flying sex workers as they are very mobile and do not do their business from one place as their counterparts who are stationed at brothels.
4. Bisexuals are men who have sex with both men and women but their predominant partners are men.
5. In fact I did not come across any study done in the hills of Darjeeling particularly, apart from a few journalistic writings.

Chapter II

Socio-Political and Economic History of Darjeeling Hills

Darjeeling developed as an urban centre when it was 'gifted' by the Rajah of Sikkim to the British as a token of friendship. Captain Llyod and Mr. Grant played an important role in getting the land which was strategically important for them. Without the recommendation of Captain Llyod and Mr. Grant, Darjeeling would have never come under the British rule. They recommended the occupation of Darjeeling as it had enormous advantages of a sanatorium and as it was strategically a very important region. The other reasons propounded by historians for the interests of the British over the region of Darjeeling are that the British wanted to 'have the safest and the shortest route to Tibet to expand trade and thwart the possible penetration of Russia, as the British efforts to open route from Nepal and Bhutan to Tibet proved hazardous' (Rai 2007). It was in January 23, 1835 that a proposal was first passed to send Captain Llyod to open negotiations with the Rajah of Sikkim for the transfer of Darjeeling to the British Government. It was later that year; that part of the present day Darjeeling was 'granted' away by the Rajah of Sikkim to the British out of friendship. 1839 was the most important year in the history of Darjeeling as the construction of the road connecting the hills and the plains was undertaken.

There were frequent violations of the Treaty of Titaliya by Sikkim under which the Rajah of Sikkim had granted Darjeeling as a gift to the British, which forced the British in 1860 to sent expeditionary forces. Following this action by the British a Treaty was concluded at Tumlong, the then capital of Sikkim. This Treaty put an end to the frontier disturbances with Sikkim and the East India Company took complete control of Darjeeling.

However, trouble arose with the adjoining state of Bhutan. "The Bhutanese were constantly engaged in aggressions on the frontier, and there was a series of outrages in which property was destroyed, lives were taken, and many innocent persons were carried off in captivity" (O'Malley 1989). Consequently, the Anglo-Bhutanese war broke out. The Bhutanese army was crushed with a heavy hand. After the war a treaty was signed by the two parties, in November 1865. Bhutan Duars with the passes leading onto the hills were ceded to the East India Company in return for an annual subsidy. Subsequently, Kalimpong was transferred to Darjeeling in 1866.

Soon after in 1866, the British undertook major developmental projects. The road from Ghoom to the plains was completed. Keeping in mind the steep gradient of this road, especially for the carts, the Darjeeling Hill Cart Road was soon constructed. This was an architectural feat of that period. The gradient of this newly built road was favourable for the construction of rail roads whose construction was also accomplished thereafter.

Building of roads and rail tracks were also results of the growing tea industry. Tea and Coffee were planted on an experimental basis. Though coffee did not show much promise, tea was found to be very suitable for the region. Soon tea became a major industry and as a result many people from neighbouring Nepal began to migrate. Tea, since then has been the mainstay of Darjeeling economy along with Timber and Tourism.

Along with tea, many other species of plants were also grown on an experimental basis. Cinchona, like tea, showed positive signs and a factory was soon set up in Mangpo. The people were quick to grasp the training they were imparted. Many new activities like copper smelting and printing were also tried but the main sources of employment remained tea and cinchona and the railway workshop at Tindharia (O'Malley 1989).

With the tea industry booming, large tracts of forestland were cleared in haste. Individual entrepreneur also tried their hands at growing tea but their experiments failed due to financial constrains. The forest supplemented the needs of the tea industry by providing timber required for making boxes to pack the manufactured tea leaves, wood-planks for construction of houses and for firewood. Keeping this in mind and the unplanned clearing of the forest the then government set up the Forest Department to look after the forest in an organized manner.

The British developed Darjeeling according to their wants and necessities. After tea, roads and railway tracks, their main concern was education. Bishop Cotton wanted to make the hills the home of European education in India and wanted to establish schools in the hills for Europeans. With his effort St. Paul's School was transferred to Darjeeling from Calcutta in 1864 (O'Malley 1989). The credit for the laying down of the infrastructure development of Darjeeling goes to the British. This has helped the people of Darjeeling tremendously.

Due to the efforts of the British, Darjeeling grew as a town. Darjeeling today is a very well known tourist spot and is also witnessing one of the fastest rates of urbanization. Over the years, the population of the area has risen tremendously.

This chapter highlights the growth of population in Darjeeling hills and in addition also gives an account of the recognized variables of HIV/AIDS like migration, intravenous drug users, alcohol use, unsafe sexual behaviour and commercial sex as is evident in the study area. Further it also brings forth the HIV/AIDS situation in the state of West Bengal and tries to locate the HIV/AIDS situation of Darjeeling in the larger picture.

Tea Plantation and Population Growth

Darjeeling saw a large number of people coming in from the neighbouring places of Nepal due to new opportunities in the tea and cinchona plantations. It was the tea plantation more than cinchona which was responsible for the growth in population. Table 2.1 illustrates the impact of tea industry on the population growth of Darjeeling district from 1861-1966.

Table 2.1: Trend in the Proportion of Tea Gardens and Work Force Participation in Darjeeling

Year	*No. of tea estates*	*Total area in hectares under tea*	*Approximate yield in kgs*	*Average yield in kgs/hectare*	*Total no. of all kinds of tea works*	*Total no. of working force*	*% of tea workers to total working force*
1861	22	1317	19323	15	2534	–	–
1871	56	–	–	–	8000	94712 (in 1872)	8.45
1881	155	11489	2340719	204	–	155779	–
1891	177	18462	4948997	268	–	155207	–
1901	170	20948	6139720	293	40451	155235	26.06
1911	156	20853	6464079	310	39561	151604	26.09
1921	168	23897	6387117	267	48710	174167	27.97
1931	169	24777	9297204	375	63665	129070	43.33
1941	136	25585	11256182	440	69699	133306	52.28
1951	138	25345	13282995	524	69590	137541	50.60
1961	145	27709	18050271	651	59844	266105	22.49
1966	144	28121	17398000	619	–	–	–

Source: A.J. Dash, Bengal District Gazetteers: Darjeeling, 1967, pp. 100.

The small hill station with a population of 100 in 1835 has now become one of the most rapidly growing urban centres. However, the main cause of the population growth has been the development of tea industry and the influx of settlers to cultivate the wastelands. As the prospects of trade and commerce grew more immigrants were again attracted. The steady improvement in communication due to the building of roads and railways along with the urbanization through the establishment of a sanatorium led to the growth of employment opportunities which subsequently led to population increase (Dewan 1991). The total population of Darjeeling along with the other sub-divisions under study is 8,30,644. In 2001, the population density of the area rose to 510, which is very high in comparison to other hill regions. Most of the population of the hills is concentrated in the sub-divisions of Darjeeling, Kalimpong and Kurseong. The sex ratio of the district is 940. There is a large variation in the sex ratio of the rural and urban areas of the sub-divisions. Today Darjeeling is witnessing a rapid pace of urbanization. The decadal growth of all the urban units *vis-a vis* Darjeeling, Kalimpong and Kurseong has been excess to 10 and Darjeeling and Kurseong has witnessed decadal growth of 46.72 and 49.56 respectively as illustrated by Table 2.2.

Migration Trends

Darjeeling grew as an urban centre under the British. Also after independence it became the district headquarters and this also facilitated its growth. As most of the government offices are located there, and having gained the reputation of being one of the most beautiful places, many people started to settle there. The growth of population was however not accompanied by a corresponding growth in infrastructure and other developments which led to the decreasing opportunities for the people. The rise in the level of education and the aspirations and fall in employment opportunities also led to large scale migration of the youth to other places, especially the metros and industrial areas. The pattern of migration has also changed. Earlier the migration of the people of Darjeeling was confined to joining the Indian army and occasionally for other government jobs. However, with the level of education among the people of Darjeeling rising, growing awareness of the outside world, decreasing employment opportunities and lack of development has led to out migration from Darjeeling. Today the youth of Darjeeling are migrating not just to join the army and to work in the informal sector but also to join MNCs and for higher studies.

The rapid urbanization in the hills resulted in the breakdown of orthodox social values, norms and customs. The joint family system which was once predominant also broke down under the pressure of the changing values, giving way to nuclear family due to employment opportunities in the towns (Lama and Chakraborty 2007). The break down of the joint family system also robbed people of the social support it provided.

The educational activities carried out by the Christian missionaries in Darjeeling witnessed a rapid growth in the number of educational institutes and also provided the people

Table 2.2: Population and Decadal Growth of Darjeeling Hills

Components of Darjeeling Hills	*Population*						*Decadal Growth Rate 1991-2001*
	1991			*2001*			
	Persons	*Male*	*Female*	*Persons*	*Male*	*Female*	
Rural Units							
Darjeeling	117196	60059	57137	115837	58407	57430	-1.16
Rangli Rangliot	65342	33367	31975	64349	32304	32045	-1.52
Kalimpong-I	53641	27445	26196	67680	34382	33298	26.17
Kalimpong-II	51411	26905	24506	60263	31309	28954	17.22
Gorubathan	46382	24203	22179	54279	27572	26707	17.03
Jorebunglow Sukiapokhri	92312	46412	45900	100724	49816	50908	9.11
Mirik	42807	22195	20612	42237	21112	21125	-1.33
Kurseong	80489	41372	39117	85867	43330	42537	6.68
Urban Units	396060	211999	184061	520432	274011	246421	31.40
Darjeeling	73062	37763	35299	107197	55963	51234	46.72
Kalimpong	38832	19973	18859	42998	22296	20702	10.73
Mirik	7022	3585	3437	9141	4619	4522	30.18
Kurseong	26758	13989	12769	40019	20410	19609	49.56

Source: Census of India 2001, Final Population Totals, West Bengal.

with the education that was helpful to aspire for the administrative jobs of the district. Today there are numerous missionary schools of repute in the hills. And along with these there are a considerable number of Government and private educational institutions though most of them are located in the towns. The institutions of Darjeeling, however, do not provide for higher education and many of the students who want to pursue higher education or technical education migrate to other places where such facilities are available. The establishment of schools by the missionaries in Darjeeling hills has provided quality primary education to the people of the hills. English has been the medium of education in a number of educational institutes. This has become helpful for the youth these days to grab the employment opportunity provided by the globalized economic structure like the call centres and other BPOs. To take advantage of this situation, a large number of young and not so young people from the hills, who are conversant in English, have joined the call centres in Delhi and other metros.

The population of Darjeeling in the early 19th century grew as many people from neighbouring areas came to work in the tea gardens. But the last decade has witnessed massive out-migration from Darjeeling because of the closure of the tea gardens, lack of employment opportunities in the government sector and the absence of private sectors in Darjeeling hills. The volume of out-migration from Darjeeling is dense.

Migration is sex selective depending on the kind of job opportunity available. Everywhere it is the young people, at the peak of their reproductive and productive health, who are the most ready to migrate. When people migrate they are dislocated from the familiar social setting which diverts from the social control and restrain one experience at the place of origin (Carballo and Siem 1996). The lack of social control, social network and the lack of awareness of safe sex and sexual health puts the migrants at the risk of STI/STD and HIV/AIDS. However, these risks are not necessarily only due to inadequate knowledge and unsafe sexual behaviour on the part of the migrants, but can also be because of the inaccessibility of health care and services to the migrants.

Most of the migrants return home during festivals and other

ceremonies. This has developed a strong circular movement among the migrants, in which the migrants move to the cities and other places of work but then make periodic visits to the families and communities. During such movements the sexual link they establish between partners in the cities and in the rural areas have the potential to develop into a significant route for HIV/AIDS transmission 'which involves families living in otherwise isolated and low risk communities' (*Ibid.*).

The spread of HIV/AIDS is closely linked to the process of migration. Migrants and mobile populations have played a significant role in the spread of HIV in the hilly regions of Darjeeling. The largely temporary character of migration in Darjeeling hills, with migrants returning home to their families on a regular basis, has facilitated the rapid spread of the virus.

Drug Abuse

Drug abuse among the people of Darjeeling was almost non-existent until the 1980s but certain indigenous substances like '*gaigure*' plant and marijuana (*ganja*) was known to the people of the hills from very early. The latter was used during certain religious festivals like '*Shivratri*.' However, the North-East drug route, frustration among the youth, lack of any creative avenues and the subsequent exposure to the world outside has facilitated the abuse of drugs in various forms in Darjeeling hills. Drug abuse is not tolerated or accepted by the society in Darjeeling hills.

Drugs abuse is prevalent in Darjeeling hills as the area is in close geographical proximity to Siliguri. Siliguri is the most important centre which connects the whole of North-East India with the rest of the country by rail and road. Trafficking of drugs from North-East India into other parts of the country takes place via Siliguri and this makes drugs easily accessible to the people of the hills. Bangladesh and Nepal borders are also very close by and there are instances of drug trafficking along these borders.

Apart from the availability of and easy access to drugs other factors have also contributed immensely to the prevalence of drug abuse in the hills. The viewing of movies in video halls in the late 80s has to a large extent contributed to the inculcation of drug habits among the youth of the hills. Movies about punk and hippie culture were very popular during that time and one of the popular video halls in Kurseong was even named 'Punk Video Hall.' Many movies were related to substance abuse. Corresponding to this period the 'Gorkhaland agitation,' for separate state and the subsequent lawlessness also facilitated drug abuse among the youth. Drug abuse and trafficking is illegal. However, during the 1980s, the police department did not prioritize the control of these activities as they were more concerned and involved in subduing the political movement. There are also conspiracy theories among the people that the police under the aegis of the state government did not pay much attention to the problem of drug abuse as they thought that the drug abusers would not be able to participate in the mass movement and the movement would get diluted in the process. Youths were also initiated into this habit by sheer curiosity and peer pressure without being aware of the risks involved.

Many of the present IDUs began with cough syrups and other tablets like N-10, Spasmoproxyvon, and Valium 10 and then started injecting intravenous drugs. Then there was a progression towards harder substances and then injecting. To save money for drugs and for bonding they started sharing needles amongst themselves. This has led to wide spread HIV infection among the IDUs in Darjeeling hills. The spread of drug addiction in the hills can be estimated from the fact that in the 5 centres of Indian Red Cross Society spread in Darjeeling hills there are 1200 IDUs registered for the Oral Substitution Therapy and Needle Syringe Exchange Programme. The nexus between substance abuse and spread of HIV/AIDS is now a well documented fact. Mode alteration associated with substance abuse leads to deviant behaviour. It further increases the chances of lifestyles where there are greater possibilities of multiple partner relations and unsafe sexual behaviour (Manderson *et al.* 2005).

Alcohol Consumption

Alcohol consumption among the people of Darjeeling is culturally prescribed. A very high percentage of the people in

Darjeeling hills consume alcohol. The relation between alcohol consumption and health is inversely proportional. This is further accentuated when there is high risk sexual behaviour under the influence of alcohol. Heavy drinkers are more likely to have unsafe sex as defined by casual associations, non-use of condoms and sex with someone who has multiple partners. In addition, men who frequently combine alcohol and sex are less likely than others, to use condoms.

Alcohol consumption among the Nepalis is culturally prescribed. The community is divided into two categories, the *'Tagedharis'* and the *'Matwalis.'* The former are culturally proscribed from consuming alcohol while for the latter alcohol forms an integral part of their culture. As the majority of the population in Darjeeling hills belong to the Nepali community, alcohol consumption is very common. Alcohol is a cultural artifact among the Nepali people; it is used during marriages, death ceremonies and child birth. Among the Rais, an ethnic group, a part of the Nepali community, alcohol is the first thing fed to a new born. As a consequence alcohol consumption in the hills is very much prevalent. The division between the *'Tagedharis'* and the *'Matwalis'* has over the years diminished because of the frequent interaction between the two groups. The earlier societal control is diffused due to a number of factors as a result of which alcohol consumption among the *Tagedharies* is increasingly prevalent.

The use of alcohol during festivals is very common and many take to consuming alcohol at a young age. There is ample evidence that a vicious progression of first alcohol and then drug addiction develops in the hills. Many of the drug addicts were first into alcohol consumption and gradually progressed into drug addiction. Even the drug addicts who want to quit drugs take up consuming alcohol.

Sex Work and Sexual Behaviour

Prostitution is an age old institution and has been prevalent in all parts of the world in different forms. Prostitution has also been practiced in Darjeeling hills from the period of early settlement. During the British rule, the deplorable conditions of the women; breaking down of marriages and also the increasing practice of prostitution in the towns was evident (Lama and Chakraborty 2007).

The traditional forms of prostitution is however not prevalent in Darjeeling. In Darjeeling there is no brothel based prostitution. As there is no brothel it is difficult to estimate the number of women engaged in this trade. The sex workers are mobile. This mobility among the sex workers has made it difficult for the agencies trying to generate awareness of HIV/AIDS and other risks involved in this trade among the FSWs. The stigma and discrimination associated with the use of sex workers stationed at the brothels is also minimized by the sex workers who are mobile. Their access to clients has also increased. People old and young are making use of the services provided by these sex workers who are less visible than their brothel based counterparts.

The growing consumerism and the lack of employment opportunities and also the irresponsible infidelity on the part of the husbands are driving many girls into this profession. Prostitution has provided an easy way to earn money and fulfil the material needs, so many are taking up this occupation.

No quantitative estimate of the practice of premarital sex is available for any rural community of India, but casual reports indicate that it is not uncommon, particularly for unmarried men. Casual sex and premarital sex among the people of Darjeeling hills have been reflected by the data collected during the field-work. There are a host of reasons why people are engaging themselves in such practices. Young boys are indulging in premarital sex to prove their masculinity whereas many girls just want to experience sex. The developments in the wider world have also affected the behavioural aspect of the people and sex which was a taboo subject for a long time has come out of the closet. Sex before marriage between boys and girls is increasing and becoming common among the youths.

Health Concerns

The district can be divided into two regions, the hilly region and the plains. The climate of the plains is hot and humid whereas the hills enjoy a pleasant climate, though the winters can be very cold. The plains were always ignored by the British and for her wonderfully bracing climate and scenic beauty Darjeeling was chosen to be developed into a sanatorium.

The topography of the region has also been instrumental in the types of health problems faced by the people. Due to heavy water-logging the plains have always faced malaria as a primary health concern. Fever was also rampant. Black water fever, kala azar locally known as *"kala dukh"*, diarrhoea, goitre and deaf mutism was common among the people, of which the latter three was more prevalent among the hill people. Small pox was also very common in the hills but the people here were not adverse to the use of vaccination (O'Malley 1989).

With time, attention was also paid to the improvement of the general health of the people. Medical institutions were slowly established. By the late 19th and early 20th century, Darjeeling had three hospitals, the Eden Sanatorium, Lowis Jubilee Sanatorium and Victoria Memorial Dispensary. The Eden Sanatorium was opened in 1883 and was meant only for the Europeans. The Lewis Jubilee Sanatorium was opened in 1887 and was meant for the natives alone. This was divided into two sections, one for the orthodox Hindus and the other for those who had no caste prejudices. The Victoria Memorial Dispensary was meant for both the Europeans and the locals (*Ibid.*).

In Kurseong, Kalimpong and many other places dispensaries were built and a large number of people were attended to every year. The Charteris Hospital in Kalimpong was maintained by the Church of Scotland Mission but aided by the State. The mission also maintained many other dispensaries. The use of *'jhankri'* (faith healers) and local medicinal plants was also prevalent at that time.

Today Darjeeling has one district hospital, two sub-divisional hospitals, two hospitals for tuberculosis, one each at Kurseong and Ghoom, and 17 primary health centres. The services provided can at best said to be mediocre. None of the hospitals are equipped to render specialized and emergency services. For any critical or complicated case the patients are referred to North Bengal Medical College and Hospital (NBMCH). The blood banks are usually without blood due to the poor storage facility. Apart from the VCCTC at the District

Hospital there are no other services provided for the control and prevention of HIV/AIDS. The Sub-Divisional Hospitals at Kalimpong and Kurseong do not cater to the needs of those infected by HIV/AIDS. However, on 'World AIDS Day' 2008 Antiretroviral Therapy (ART) centre was inaugurated at the District Hospital and ICTC centres in the two Sub-Divisional Hospitals at Kalimpong and Kurseong were also started in the early 2009.

HIV/AIDS Scenario in Darjeeling Hills

Though West Bengal is considered a low prevalence state, it is highly vulnerable. West Bengal has been characterized as a low prevalence state because the median prevalence is below 1 per cent for ANC sites and below 5 per cent in STD clinic sites. Presently a few hot spots indicate a raging concentrated epidemic in the state, which are Kolkata and its suburbs, and the urban areas of the adjoining districts of Howrah and Hoogly, North & South 24-Parganas and Haldia. The epidemic seems to be more significant among the lower socio-economic groups mostly comprising of migrants (WBSAP&CS 2006). Among the High Risk population West Bengal showed decreasing trend in all the groups other than MSM group where the prevalence rate increased from 0.54 in 2005 to 6.6 per cent in 2006. The HIV prevalence rate among the ANC cases remains somewhere at 0.4 per cent over the years. HIV prevalence in STD that year stood at 1.66 per cent down from 2.79 per cent in 2004 and 2.47 per cent in 2005. HIV prevalence in FSW has gone down from 6.8 per cent to 6.6 per cent and prevalence in IDUs decreased to 4.64 per cent from 7.41 per cent; only MSM component has seen an upward trend in the 10th round of surveillance where prevalence rate shoot up from 0.54 per cent to 6.12 per cent (WBSAP&CS 2007)

In Darjeeling hills the prevalence of HIV/AIDS appears to be low, however, it is a major public health issue as it has been recognized by NACO as a very vulnerable area. The first case of HIV/AIDS in Darjeeling was identified in 2002, in an'IDU after the setting up of the VCCTC at the Eden Hospital. Since then the number of people infected and affected has gradually increased. Till November 2007, the total number of HIV/AIDS cases had reached 141 in Darjeeling hills. The total number of men infected is 93 and the number of females infected is 43 and 5 are children. This rapid increase of the disease is also likely to be underreported partly because of the paucity of HIV/AIDS surveillance centres and the inadequacy of testing centres. Furthermore, the varying latency of HIV/AIDS among people suggests that some HIV/AIDS infected individuals may not manifest the symptoms for months or even years, even though they can transmit the virus to others. As one doctor said, *"The number is just a tip of an iceberg. The number can be ten folds more. Due to the lack of awareness and the inaccessibility of the VCCTC many are unable to get themselves tested. Again the well to do people does not get tested here as they fear the consequences of being positive. Therefore in all likelihood the number of positive people in the hills can be much higher than what is presented by the VCCTC data."*

The demography of the reported HIV/AIDS cases in Darjeeling hills indicates that approximately two-third of those infected are males. The infection is most prevalent in the 20-39 years age group among both the sexes. The predominant mode of transmission is heterosexual sex, sharing of needles among IDUs and migration. A doctor from Kalimpong said, *"Here in the hills there are many reasons for the spread of the infections. People these days are engaging in casual sex and drugs addiction is also very high. The migrants are also responsible for the spread of this infection. Many join the army and bring the infection. In Kalimpong alone we have found 7 cases among the military people. Alcoholism is a major cause. As girls are easily available and after drinking people want to have sex. People do not have much knowledge about prevention of this infection. We can also say that the social changes taking place is also fuelling the spread of HIV/AIDS."*

The HIV/AIDS cases have seen a gradual rise in the hills since the inception of VCCTC. In the first year, the number of cases detected was 7. Every year there was a rise in the number of cases and only in the 2004 was there a marginal decline, when only 17 cases were detected. The yearly figures from 2002 to 2007 are shown in Fig. 2.1.

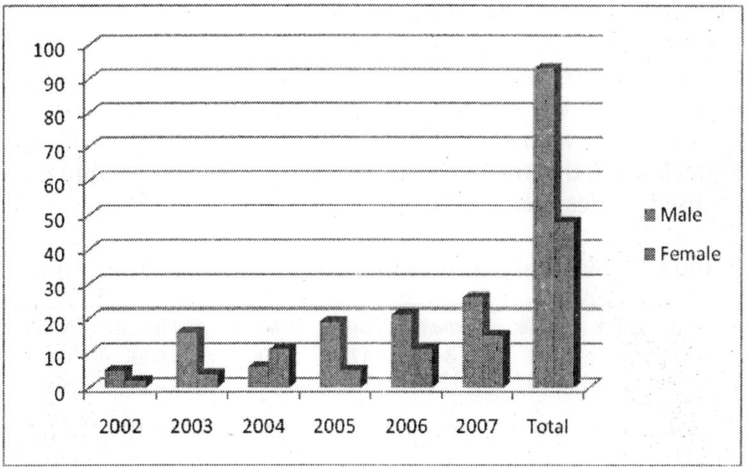

Fig. 2.1: Yearly Infection in Darjeeling Hills, 2002-07

Source: Darjeeling VCCTC, Eden Hospital, Darjeeling.

Large number of PLWHA is married and reportedly many are those who have been working outside Darjeeling. Till now there have been 2276 tests done in the VCCTC and the positivity rate is 6.19 per cent. The prevalence rate is 0.03. The per cent of positivity among those coming to VCCTC suggests that if proper surveillance is done then the number can go very high as many people do not have access to VCCTC as there is only one in the area. The VCCTC is also not equipped properly to handle the large number of cases that are being detected. As the hospital do not provide for any other services apart from testing and counselling most of the people who are found to be positive are asked to go to Shanker Foundation—a network of positive people, which maintains records of its members, for further counselling, care and support.

For this analysis members of Shanker Foundation have been taken into consideration. There have been 17 deaths reported by Shanker Foundation due to HIV/AIDS. However, all those who are tested are not its members. Many chose not to be its member fearing stigma and discrimination. These reported deaths are the records of its registered members only. Today the total number of members of Shanker Foundation is 56. The members comprise of 34 male, 22 female. Among them there are 4 children. Among the members 39 were ever married, 20 male and 19 female. There were relatively a large proportion of widows in the members of the Foundation. Among the 19 ever married women members 6 were widows (31.6%) which suggests that the burden of the disease is being invariably faced by the females (Table 2.3).

Table 2.3: Marital Status of Members of Shanker Foundation

Marital Status	*Male*	*Female*	*Total*	*% Male*	*% Female*	*% Total*
Single	14	3	17	25.00	5.35	30.35
Married	19	13	32	33.92	23.21	57.13
Divorcee	1	0	1	1.78	0	1.78
Widow(er)	0	6	6	0	10.71	10.71
Total	34	22	56	60.70	39.27	99.97

Source: Shanker Foundation, Darjeeling.

The oldest among the male members of Shanker Foundation is 44 years old and the youngest is 5 years old and the oldest female is 39 years old and the youngest is 7 years old. The majority among both the male and female come within the 21-39 age groups. However, the educational background and income of the members was not available (Table 2.4).

Table 2.4: Age Structure of the Members of Shanker Foundation

Age Group	*Male*	*Female*	*Total*
5-20	3	1	4
21-25	6	6	12
26-30	5	4	9
31-35	9	5	14
36-40	8	6	14
41-45	3	0	3
46-50	0	0	0
Total	34	22	56

Source: Shanker Foundation, Darjeeling.

Darjeeling has been identified as the most vulnerable to HIV/AIDS by WBSAC&PS. HIV/AIDS has already entered most of the high risk groups and can spread to the general population as multiple sexual partners is common and people do not have a very comprehensive knowledge about HIV/AIDS, its prevention and treatment. The risk of HIV/AIDS in the hills is succinctly described by the convener of one of the NGOs in Darjeeling. He said, *"People do not have much idea about the infection and lack awareness and knowledge about it. Here the prevalence rate is 0.5-6.6. The prevalence of HIV due to sexual activities is 86 per cent and from blood transfusion is 2 per cent."*

It is clear that the advent of HIV/AIDS in Darjeeling will be a greater cause of worry for the government as the health infrastructure and the corresponding facilities are not sufficient to confront the epidemic. The socio-economic conditions of the people are also not very good so that the people in the absence of any ART centre can procure the medicine on their own and look after themselves. The spread of the epidemic will see the administration of the area ill-prepared to tackle it. The next chapter gives a detailed analysis of the socio-demographic profile of the study population.

Chapter III

Socio-Demographic Profile of the Study Population

This chapter deals with the socio-demographic conditions of the sample population and also analyses in detail each category of the groups of people that make up the sample population. The chapter highlights the age structure, educational qualification, income etc. of the sample population. The chapter also profiles the PLWHA and highlights their different experiences.

Population Composition

The sample is based on a number of variables like age, religion, gender, education and income. The size of the sample is 210. There are 31 key informants, comprising mostly of doctors and NGO personnels.[1] The sample is predominantly male as many of the females who were approached for interview did not want to talk about HIV/AIDS. The sample can be categorized as community members, Flying Sex Workers (FSWs), Intravenous Drug Users (IDUs), bisexuals[2] and caregivers. The male (139) comprise approximately 66 per cent of population. The female (71) comprise approximately 34 per cent. Among the community members, which make 73.3 per cent of the sample, 20 per cent are female. Among the PLWHA who comprise 5.2 per cent of the sample population, 3.3 per cent are female. The FSWs who make 9.0 per cent of the sample are all female.

Among the IDUs, there are 1.5 per cent female and among the bisexuals there are no female (Table 3.1). The numbers of bisexuals in the sample is 9 and are also included in the total number of male. The predominance of male in the sample can be attributed to the fact that they were not hesitant to talk about HIV/AIDS and their personal sexual behaviour.

Table 3.1: The Composition of the Sample Population

Category	*Male*	*Female*	*Total*	*% Male*	*% Female*	*%Tota*
Community Members	112	42	154	53.33	20.0	73.33
PLWHA	4	7	11	1.90	3.33	5.23
FSWS	0	19	19	0.0	9.05	9.05
IDU	14	3	17	6.67	1.43	8.10
Bisexuals	9	0	9	4.29	0.0	4.29
Total	139	71	210	66.19	33.81	100

Source: Field Data.

Religion

The sample is diverse in terms of religion. The majority of them are Hindus (104) followed by Buddhists (59), Christians (43) and Muslims (4). The Hindus comprise 49.51 per cent of the sample population. The Buddhists comprise 28.08 per cent, the Christians comprise 20.46 per cent and the Muslims 1.89 per cent of the sample respectively. Table 3.2 illustrates the religious composition of the sample population.

Table 3.2: Religious Composition of the Sample Population

Religion	*Male*	*Female*	*Total*	*% Male*	*% Female*	*% Total*
Hindu	80	24	104	38.09	11.42	49.51
Buddhist	29	30	59	13.80	14.28	28.08
Christians	27	16	43	12.85	7.61	20.46
Muslims	3	1	4	1.42	0.48	1.90
Total	139	71	210	66.19	33.81	100.00

Source: Field Data.

Age Structure

The age structure of the sample is varied. The youngest among the sample population is 18 years old and the oldest is 48 years old. The majority of the sample falls under the group of 26-30 years and comprises 34.7 per cent. 21-25 years of age group comprises 34.2 per cent of the sample. The least number of the sample falls under the age group of 41-45 years and is only 1 in number. The largest number of men falls under the age group of 26-30 years and comprises 33.8 per cent of their total. The largest number of women falls under the age group of 21-25 years and comprises 43.6 per cent of their total. The least number of women fall under the age group of 36-40 years (Table 3.3).

Table 3.3: Age Structure of the Sample Population

Age Group	Male	Female	Total	% Male	% Female	% Total
16-20	27	3	30	12.86	1.43	14.29
21-25	41	31	72	19.52	14.76	34.28
26-30	47	26	73	22.38	12.38	34.76
31-35	12	10	22	5.71	4.76	10.47
36-40	8	1	9	3.81	0.48	4.29
41-45	1	0	1	0.48	0.0	0.48
46-50	3	0	3	1.43	0.0	1.43
Total	139	71	210	66.19	33.81	100.00

Source: Field Data.

Education

The literacy rate of Darjeeling district is at par with the national literacy rate. Only one respondent was found to be illiterate. The highest educational qualification of the sample population is M.A. There are four respondents who hold a masters degree and there are 79 who hold a bachelors degree. There are 61 respondents who have completed their education up to class XII and 31 have completed their education up to class X level. 34 respondents have attended school but have failed to complete class X. 42.2 per cent of the female respondents are graduates. There is also a high number of female respondents who have completed their studies up to class XII (Table 3.4).

The female literacy rate of the district is higher than that of the national average. Most of the sample population has completed education up to the matric level.

Table 3.4: Education Level of the Sample Population

Sex	*PG*	*Graduate*	*UG*	*Class X*	*Below X*	*Illiterate*	*Total*
Male	4	49	51	25	10	0	139
Female	0	30	10	6	24	1	71
Total	4	79	61	31	34	1	210

Source: Field Data.

Marital Status

The largest portion of the sample is single men and women. The single men comprise 35.71[3] per cent of the sample and the women comprise 19.5 per cent of the sample. The married men comprise 29 per cent and the women falling under this category is 10.5 per cent of the sample. Of all who are divorced 1.4 per cent is men and 1.0 per cent is female respectively. Widows comprise 2.9 per cent of the sample (Table 3.5). Divorced and widowed female fall under the category of FSWs and PLWHA.

Table 3.5: Marital Status of the Sample Population

Marital Status	*Male*	*Female*	*Total*	*% Male*	*% Female*	*(%) Total*
Single	75	41	116	35.71	19.52	55.23
Married	61	22	83	29.05	10.48	39.53
Divorced	3	2	5	1.43	0.95	2.38
Widow	0	6	6	0	2.86	2.86
Total	139	71	210	66.19	33.81	100.00

Source: Field Data.

Work Status and Income

Most of the sample population is self-employed. The number of people doing business is 57 and forms 27.1 per cent of the sample. Among the category of self-employed the FSWs are also included. There are 36 government employees in the sample and they form 17.1 per cent of the sample. Most of the government employees earn more than rupees 7500 per month. Among the casual workers who form 17.2 per cent of the sample the largest number falls under the Rs. 3000-5000 per month range. The labour category has the least representation and constitutes only 2.8 per cent of the sample population. However, unemployed people constitute the largest number of the sample population and represents 35.7 per cent of the sample (Table 3.6).

Table 3.6: Work Status and Income

Work Status	*Number (%)*	*Income*	*Number*
Govt. Service[4]	36 (17.2)	<3000	6
		3000-5000	5
		5001-7500	6
		7500+	19
Business[5]	57 (27.1)	<3000	13
		3000-5000	27
		5001-7500	9
		7500+	8
Casual Service[6]	36 (17.2)	<3000	8
		3000-5000	24
		5001-7500	0
		7500+	4
Labour[7]	6 (2.8)	<3000	1
		3000-5000	5
		5001-7500	0
		7500+	0
Unemployed[8]	75 (35.7)	Not Applicable	75
Total	210 (100)		210

Source: Field Data.

PLWHA in Darjeeling Hills

Traditional approaches to the life cycle of human beings have tended to assume a fairly predictable progression through a sequence of life stages, from birth to death via childhood, marriage and old age. Society has been managing this transition from one stage to another successfully. However, this is an idealized pattern of life cycle. But there are differences between the idealized and the real life, especially in today's postmodern world. There is a breakdown of traditional beliefs and practices and there is a rise in individualism which forces individuals to take risks and make choices. Several important life transitions—sexual initiation, partnership formation, leaving school, childbearing and entering into labour force—takes place by the time an individual reaches the second decade of his/her life. Today in an individualistic consumerist society there are impediments which individuals have to face and negotiate in their lives. HIV/AIDS is not only one of the most salient barriers in today's world for an individual to develop oneself as a complete human being but is also a risk in making choices. While individualism is an important aspect of today's life, the individual is part of the society, and the product of social structures and processes which make the society. Their education, their sexual and reproductive behaviour, their readiness to take the role and responsibility of adulthood and the support they receive from the families and communities and government will determine their own futures. HIV/AIDS can also be viewed as a product of complex social structures and processes rather than the simple result of individual behaviour.

Studies on HIV/AIDS have proved this view and have been to a large extent enriched by the writings and life experiences of PLWHA. Their accounts have become politically meaningful and powerful because they have helped us understand and challenge disabling obstacles. They have been helpful because they enable us to understand more about the ways in which they work and how PLWHA have challenged social relations. This section tries to investigate and examine the lived experiences of the PLWHA and how they are challenging the situation in Darjeeling.

The PLWHA in Darjeeling hills are a hidden populations. They are hidden because of their infection which is very often stigmatized and discriminated (Simbayi *et al.* 2007), and those infected by the disease have not yet had the courage to disclose their status to the outside world. They have lost their social dignity as they are seen as deviant and wrong doers. Table 3.7 illustrates the characteristics of the PLWHA who are also the constituents of the sample.

There were 4 males and 7 females PLWHA in the sample which were studied. The females were more in number because they were usually present in the office of Shanker Foundation. The salient modes of transmission of HIV/AIDS in Darjeeling

Table 3.7: Characteristics of the PLWHA

Characteristics	*Male*	*%*	*Female*	*%*	*Total*
Transmission					
Homosexual	0	0	0	0	0
Heterosexual	1	9.09	7	63.63	72.72
IDU	3	27.27	0	0	27.27
Blood Transfusion	0	0	0	0	0
Employment Status					
Employed	3	27.27	2	18.18	45.45
Unemployed	1	9.09	5	45.45	54.54
Living Arrangement					
Alone	0	0	0	0	0
With Wife/Husband	1	9.09	1	9.09	18.18
With Parents and Others	3	27.27	6	54.54	81.81
Age in Years					
<20	0	0	0	0	0
21–40	4	36.36	7	63.63	99.99
>40	0	0	0	0	0

Source: Field Data.

hills are heterosexual intercourse and sharing of infected needles. There are also cases of Parent to Child Transmission. There are no reported cases of other forms of transmission among the PLWHA who were part of the study. All but one male respondent were infected because of needle sharing and comprised 27.27 per cent while the female respondents were infected by the heterosexual intercourse and comprised of 63.63 per cent. All the female respondents except one who was single at the time of interview were infected through heterosexual intercourse and by their husbands. There were no other forms of transmission reported by the respondents. All the respondents fall under the age group of 21-40 (Table 3.7). The absence of the other forms of transmission can be attributed to many factors as one of the employees of Shanker Foundation tried to rationalize and said, "*There is not much evidence of other forms of transmission here as the men who have sex with men are a hidden population and are not high in number. Firstly, they may not know that they are infected because of their isolation and unwillingness to mix up with others. Secondly, even if they know they will not come and say it to the people around as they are so much ridiculed because of their sexual preferences and their physical conditions. The absence of those who are infected due to blood transfusion are not known as they are mostly infected outside Darjeeling and are generally from the upper strata of the society and would not like to disclose their identity and status and be involved with the members of Shanker Foundation. Further many do not know about this organization as well. The primary reason for many people not coming to Shanker Foundation is also because of the lack of knowledge of HIV/AIDS among the people."*

Of the 4 male respondents 3 were employed by Shanker Foundation as volunteers and as peer educator. The female respondents were also employed as volunteers by the organization. However, their salary was a paltry sum given to them as a token of gratitude. The salary did not matter to them as this provided them with an opportunity to engage in something and forget their personal trauma. As one of the female respondents said, *"The work I do here gives me immense satisfaction as I am doing something for our community and I get to spend lot of time with people who are facing similar problems like I do and are going through the same ordeals. So working here is not about money but the support we generate for each other."*

There were no respondents living alone and the majority was living with their parents and other members of the family. As most of the females were widows they were being looked after by someone or the other from either her husband's or her own family's side. The one single female respondent who was staying with her parents had however not disclosed her sero positive status to her parents at the time of interview. There were two, a male and a female respondent, who were living with their wife and husband respectively. However, one was a discordant couple and the wife had already had herself tested and was asked to undergo another test after six months.

All the respondents were in the economically productive age group of 21-40. The oldest among the male respondents was 38 years old and among the female respondents was a 37 year old and undergoing antiretroviral therapy. She reported living with her family members though at the time of the interview she was living at the Glen Foundation, Kalimpong. 7 of the respondents were in the age group of 23-29 and the rest four were in the age group of 30-38. There were three respondents who were married and comprised of 27.27 per cent and there were two respondents who were single and comprised of 18.18 per cent. There was only one respondent who was divorced and the majorities of the respondents were widows (5) and comprised of 45.45 per cent of the PLWHA's sample (Tables 3.8 and 3.9).

Table 3.8: Marital Status and Educational Qualification of the PLWHA

Characteristics	*Frequency (n=11)*
Marital Status	
Married	3
Single	2
Widow	5
Divorced	1
Educational Qualification	
B.A.	0
Class 12	4
Class 10	2
< Class 10	4
Never Attended School	1
Time of Being Diagnosed as HIV positive	4 months-5 years

Source: Field Data.

Table 3.9: Time since Infection was Diagnosed among PLWHA

Sl. No	*Sex*	*Age*	*Time Since Positive*
1	M	38	5 years
2	M	32	1 year
3	M	25	4 months
4	M	24	7 months
5	F	30	3 years 4 months
6	F	25	1 year 6 months
7	F	28	4 years
8	F	23	4 months
9	F	37	4 years 6 months
10	F	29	9 months
11	F	27	6 months

Source: Field Data.

Among the nine married respondents, 6 have children. Three of the children were tested and two of them were found to be HIV sero negative while the one living with a widowed mother is sero positive. Three parents reported not to have tested their children at the time of interview. The fear of not being able to face the situation if the child was found to be positive has stopped them from getting their children tested.

The respondents are educated but their education level is not very high. The maximum respondents have studied up to class 12 and there is one respondent who has never attended school. There are 4 respondents who have completed high school and comprises of 36.36 per cent. One respondent has completed matriculation and the rest are school drop-outs. Overall the respondents belong to the lower socio-economic strata.

The respondents were all tested in Darjeeling and their CD4 was counted in NBMCH, at Siliguri. 63.63 per cent of the respondents had a high CD4 count as a consequence they were not undergoing ART whereas 36.36 per cent were undergoing ART. They were receiving the ART from NBMCH and one respondent also reported getting ART from Glen Foundation, Kalimpong. Among the respondents receiving ART, 3 (27.27%) were female and only 1 (9.09%) was male. Three (27.27%) respondents had opportunistic infection (OI) at the time of interview and all of them were female.

Experiences of Positive People

First Thoughts on Being HIV Positive

All the PLWHA remembered vividly the day they were tested and also the first thought that came to their mind on hearing that they were positive. The respondents reported not to have known much about the disease, HIV/AIDS, before they were asked to go for the test and visit the VCCTC. Only a handful among them had heard that HIV/AIDS spreads through sexual intercourse and that it would happen only to the *'morally bad people.'* This misconception about the infection gave them a false hope that they were not vulnerable and susceptible to it after their repeated exposure to the dangers of getting infected. All the female respondents reported that they had never imagined even in their dreams that they would be infected by HIV/AIDS. As one female respondent said, *"I had never in my dreams thought that I would get this disease as I had no bad habits. I was married when I was young. I always thought that only the 'bad girls' would get this disease. But today I am infected with it. What can I do? I could not believe that I was diagnosed to be positive. Even when I was going for the test I thought that it cannot happen to me."* Another respondent said, *"When I was advised by the doctor treating my husband that I should get tested for HIV/AIDS I was offended and argued with the doctor and swore at him as I thought that it could happen only to the 'bad people' but the doctor was right and I was diagnosed to be positive."* Another respondent said, *"HIV/AIDS never leaves anybody if you are not careful. I was of the opinion that it could not happen to me but I am positive today."*

The male respondents also thought that they were not vulnerable to HIV/AIDS and their behaviour was not prone to it. One of the male respondents said, *"When I was doing drugs I never thought that I would be HIV positive someday. In fact I did not know about it and HIV/AIDS was not known in Darjeeling then. I was sick when the doctor told me to get tested. I wondered why the doctor was asking me to get HIV/AIDS test done. I told him that I had never had sex outside marriage but then the doctor said that IDUs were also very susceptible to HIV/AIDS. To my knowledge I am the first to get tested for HIV/AIDS and diagnosed positive in the entire Darjeeling hills. If only I had known that even sharing needles would make one vulnerable to HIV/AIDS then I would not have married."* Another male respondent said, *"When my parents came to know that I was into drugs they decided to send to Kripa[9] for detoxification. During my stay there I learnt about HIV/AIDS and was very nervous and scared. I did give up drugs while I was in Kripa. Soon I was released and when I came home I did not go out for months. Once my mother asked me to go out and not spent so much time at home. Then I started going out and soon I was into drugs again. So again they sent me to Kripa. There some HIV/AIDS prevention programme was going on and I was asked to do the test. I was sure that I would not be infected and did the test and was found to be infected. Even after doing the test three times I could not believe that I was positive. Had I known earlier that injecting was such a fatal thing then maybe I would not have done it but then there was not much knowledge about it."* Another male respondent said, *"I did not know much about HIV/AIDS when I was infected. If only I knew that the use of condom would protect one from the infection then probably I would be HIV negative now."* A female respondent said, *"I did not know about HIV/AIDS when I was found to be infected with it. Still I do not understand much about it as I am illiterate. However, even if I had the knowledge about it, I would not have been able to protect myself from it as I was infected by my husband. If he had known about HIV/AIDS then both of us would had been safe and healthy now."*

Most of the respondents still remembered their first thought as the news of their sero status reached them. As most of them were of the opinion that they could never be infected by HIV/AIDS and it was news of shock and disbelief. However, the thought of parents was prominent among the respondents. Ten of the respondents said that they were in a state of denial and could not trust the test and actually thought that may be some mistake had occurred with the test. The incurable nature of HIV/AIDS frightened most of the respondents and many anticipated death when they were diagnosed to be HIV positive. Some of the male respondents however show some resentment for their behaviour.

One of the respondents said, *"When the result of my blood test was given to me I did not understand and asked the doctor to explain it to me. When he said that I was HIV/AIDS positive I was shocked and thought that may be there was something wrong with the result and told the doctor that it may not be my report. However, when the doctor said that it was my report and that I was actually HIV positive, I could not think of what I would do in life for a while. I thought that I may die soon"* Another respondent said, *"I could not think of anything except death at the time of receiving the report of my blood test. I thought that I must be the most useless character in this whole world as I had troubled my parents throughout and did nothing apart from doing drugs and did not obey my parents. Only if I had listened to them I would not be in this situation."* Another male respondent said, *"When I went to collect my report I was told that I was HIV positive. I did not understand the enormity of the situation properly. Only after I could gather everything that was told during the time of counselling did I realize what it meant to be HIV sero positive. I thought I would soon be dying and would leave my parents. I thought that it was the consequences of my behaviour. When the whole world had asked me to give up drugs I had always cheated by saying that I will give up and never made any effort at quitting it.*

Then I thought about the guys with whom I had shared needles and felt very bad for them." Another male respondent who was infected through heterosexual intercourse said, *"At the time when I came to know about my sero status I was nervous and shocked. For a while I could not think of anything. I had the report on one hand and I was trembling. I thought that I was on the doorsteps of death. I thought of where could I have gone wrong and where did I get infected. I thought of all the places where I had had sex with different girls. Only after a while did I think about my wife and my parents. I thought that I have to leave them on their own and what will they do to lead their life without me."*

The female respondents were shocked as well. Their narratives reflect the intersection of death and their concern for their family. One of the respondents said, *"I was pregnant when I was advised to the test. When I got the report I was shocked to know that I was positive. I knew then that I was going to die soon. However, I was more concerned about the unborn baby as to whether or not it would be positive. I just could not imagine that an unborn baby could be infected with such a deadly disease and die without being able to see the world."* Another respondent said, *"When I was called to collect my report I was a bit nervous but confident that I could never be HIV positive but when I collected the report the confidence turned into shock. I thought that the whole world was tumbling down upon me. I sat on the floor and thought what I will do now with this disease, which is not going to be cured. I thought about everybody I knew and everybody who knew me. I thought about my old in-laws."* Another respondent said, *"I thought that I would never be infected with HIV/AIDS. When I received the report I was flabbergasted. I could not believe that I was positive. I became hysterical, I cried and laughed. I just thought that I would now die within a short period and that my child would be alone. I thought that I was innocent and was not to be blamed about this condition. I thought that many people would blame me and level me a bad character woman. There were so many thoughts at that time."* Another respondent said, *"It was shocking to hear that I was HIV positive. I wanted to kill myself on hearing that I was positive. However, the thought of my husband and other people I love stopped me. Even many days after knowing my sero status I thought of committing suicide but I could not."* Another respondent said, *"I could not believe that I was positive so I abused the doctor. Then I realized that this was my fate. I cried on the shoulders of the doctor. I thought that my days were numbered and I would die soon."* The only female respondent who was single at the time of interview said, *"I did not believe that I was positive. I cried a lot. I wanted to die there and not return home but I thought of my parents who are very fond of me and somehow left the hospital. I cried and cried for many days and did not do anything. Till the time I came to know about Shanker Foundation I had been crying."* Another female respondent said, *"I could not believe that I was positive. I was shocked, ashamed and scared that I would die soon. It was like the end of my life. I could not think of anything apart from death."*

Reactions of the PLWHA's about the Source of Infection

None of the female respondents thought about the person who infected them with this fatal virus at the time of knowing their sero status. When the researcher asked them about the person who infected them they said that they had no ill feeling towards the infector, but only at times of depression and desperation did they feel that their partners should have been honest and not transmitted the virus to them. The only single female respondent in the sample said, *"I did not think about my boy friend immediately when I knew about my sero status. When I thought about him, initially I thought that I will ruin him by telling everybody that he is HIV positive as I am sure he is, otherwise I would not have been positive. Then I thought that may be, he does not know. It is the result of his bad behaviour. I do not have to curse him as he will suffer as much as I have to."* However, the widows were in fact, missing their husbands who were their infectors. One of the widows said, *"I will not curse my husband as he is already dead. We should pray for the departed soul. I do feel bad and cheated when I think that he transmitted the virus to me but I miss him and wish he was alive and sharing the difficulties I face today."* Another widow said, *"I don't think he did it knowingly. If he had known that I would be infected by him then I think he would not have done it. I only wish he had not got into drugs."* Another widow said, *"Maybe it was my fault that I would not take good care of him. Otherwise he would not have visited all those places and got himself infected. I do get angry when I think about him but again he was my husband and wish he is at peace."* Another widow said, *"I don't know how he could have done this to me. I trusted and loved him so much. I even married him against the wishes of my parents and this is what I get for loving him. I just hate him for what he has done to me. However, I do not know how to react most of the times. When I think of him and the time we spent together as the most pleasant memories of my life, are connected with him. I only hope he was alive and helping me to face this adversity."* The only married female respondent who was not a widow at the time of the interview said, *"If he was honest with me this would not have happened. Even after I got married I did not know that he was married earlier and his first wife had passed away. Even his parents did not tell me. I think he wanted somebody to share his difficulties and grievances so maybe he married me. He may have his reasons but I just loath him for what he has done."*

The male respondents did not think about the persons who may have been responsible for transmitting the virus to them and were even sensible in not blaming their colleagues with whom they *'fixed'* together. They were just contemplating about the life ahead and thinking of the inevitable death that would follow HIV/AIDS. One respondent who believes himself to be among the first to be tested and found to be infected and publicly disclose his status in the Darjeeling hills said, *"I do not know how this virus entered Darjeeling and our lives and do not blame anybody for bringing it here. It can be anybody as there were a number of guys who used to go to other places and get their 'fix' as I have also done. So it is irrelevant to blame others. I am just concerned that there may be many more there with the virus but do not know about it and are posing a danger to many others. It is therefore important to get them tested. The fear of HIV/AIDS is such that people are scared to get themselves tested. These days I just think that the Shanker Foundation becomes empowered and financially sound so that we can take care of all the PLWHA and lead an exemplary life."* Another respondent who was also infected because of intravenous drug use said, *"I do not care who infected me or how I was infected. It is already too late for me to think about all these things. I just hope I can live a healthy life now and help others. I just want to repent for my past life and behaviour. I want to help as many people as possible and protect them from HIV/AIDS. This has now become my concern as well as goal in life."* Another respondent said, *"I never thought of the guys I 'hanged' around with or shared 'fixes' when I was diagnosed with HIV. I was just too concerned about myself and the life I would have and the death that would follow. I do not know if I got infected because some of my acquaintances were already infected and do not have anything against them as we did everything together knowingly and unknowingly. We did not know about HIV/AIDS so there is no point in blaming them or just doubting them for my infection. I pray to God and hope that my friends did not get the infection from me. If my friends are negative than I think that my prayers are answered."*

Concern of the PLWHA for Disclosing their Status

As the respondent who was tested in 2002 said, *"At the time of my diagnosis there was not much knowledge about HIV/AIDS and subsequently the stigma and discrimination associated with it. I did not know what to do then as I only knew that I would be dying soon. The doctor called me to his office and told me not to talk about this disease with anyone. So I did not disclose my status to anybody. I think if the doctor had not stopped me maybe I would have disclosed my status and the fear of people regarding HIV/AIDS might have lessened by now."* Another female respondent said, *"I was asked by the doctors to get the HIV test done after my husband was found to be HIV positive. He was very ill and died soon. I tested and when my result came the doctor disclosed that I was positive in the presence of my sister-in-law. I did not have any choice but to tell the other family members as well that I was positive. If the doctor had not disclosed it in her presence then I would not have disclosed it to anybody."* The narratives of these two PLWHA show that they had no control over the issue of disclosure of their sero status. The respondent's right to share or not to share their sero status and the issue of confidentiality was taken away by the doctors. The respondent's anger against the doctors is evident. However, the fact that nothing could had been done against them is also clear as the female respondent said, *"I could not do anything against the doctor for disclosing the sero status in front of my sister-in-law. I did not know anything regarding HIV/AIDS and at that time just wanted to live longer. The important thing at that time for me was that I was under the supervision of that doctor and the only thing I knew then was that he would help me to live some days more. I was too dependent on him. So I thought that seeking reasons for his disclosure and telling him that it was unnecessary, will not do any good to me."* The anger towards the erroneous doctor, the feeling of resignation and the feeling that doctors were the ones who could help them live a little longer and going against them was futile is evident from the above narrative.

The majority of the respondents have disclosed their status according to their convenience. Most of the respondents had not disclosed their status to the public due to fear of discrimination and isolation. Keeping their positive status a secret gave a great sense of relief and strength to the PLWHA and some of the respondents were of the opinion that their immediate concern was to keep their status as discreet as possible. Discrimination was the main reason for not disclosing their status. One of the respondents said, *"There are only five of us in the whole region who have disclosed the sero status to the public. Not disclosing the status was torturing us and we also wanted to prove that people can live a normal life with the virus and educate people on HIV/AIDS. The discriminating nature of the disease has kept many people away from Shanker Foundation. We want them to come to Shanker Foundation and increase our strength so that we can work together for our betterment. We want to tell them as well as the public that there is life beyond HIV/AIDS."*

Another respondent said, *"I have not disclosed my status to anybody apart from my sister-in-law. I stay with her, she is very helpful and caring I don't have to fear that she will disclose my status I do not want to disclose it to anybody as people are still scared of HIV/AIDS and discriminates us. I am happy now and can walk around without any fear of discrimination. Other members of Shanker Foundation want us to disclose our status so that we can put some pressure on the people who are responsible for our welfare but I will only disclose my status when I think the time is right."* Another respondent said, *"I am still not in the right frame of mind to disclose my status. It has just been 4 months since my diagnosis and am still trying to cope with the consequences of the disease, so I don't want to disclose my sero status. When I think I can take all the hardship associated with the infection then I will disclose my status."* Another respondent said, *"I will only disclose my positive status to very close persons and that too if I think that they will not discriminate or hate me for the infection. Otherwise I will not disclose it. It is very difficult to stay the way I am staying today. I keep myself away from everybody as I fear I may transmit the virus somehow to the others so*

I try to isolate myself from the rest of the society. I just hate to be in isolation but what to do, there is no other way out. When the society accepts us then I will disclose my status." Another respondent said, *"It is not easy to stay this way hiding from everybody but this is the best I can do to my child. He goes to school and if it is known that I am positive then they will also come to know about his status. I have to keep my positivity a secret to save my child from the society and discrimination. My parents are also old and they look after both of us but they will not be able to face the discrimination. What will happen when they are ill? No one will come to help and support us if they know that we are both positive. I do not intend to disclose my sero positive status but don't know what will happen in the future as these guys are doing so much for the members here so maybe I will also disclose my status and help with their work outside Shanker Foundation."* Another respondent said, *"I will try to make a right decision regarding disclosing my status. I have always made the wrong decisions in life and for once I would like to make a correct decision which will be beneficial to everybody."* Another respondent says, *"Regarding the disclosure of my status to the public I will take as much time as possible. Now only the family knows and at times it is very scary to think that they might just let the world know about it. I will declare myself when I think the time is right."*

One male respondent said, *"Among the people here the kinship bonding is quite strong. Even cousins are in regular touch with one another. At times of happiness and sorrow the strength of such bonds is evident. Under such circumstances it is impossible to keep the diagnosis a secret."*

The public fear surrounding HIV/AIDS as well as their moral judgment makes it difficult for the PLWHA of Darjeeling to come out in the society and disclose their positive status.

PLWHA's Experiences in the Health Care Settings

The experiences of the PLWHA in the health setting are not positive as they have to face a number of problems. The health officials in many parts of India are not well aware and well informed about HIV/AIDS and its treatment, especially those in the lower rungs of the hierarchy (*www.avert.org.*), so is the case in Darjeeling. A retired senior doctor from a public hospital, currently working in a private hospital in India had said, *"There is an almost hysterical kind of fear…at all levels, starting from the humblest, the sweeper or the ward boy, up to the heads of departments, which makes them pathologically scared of having to deal with an HIV-positive patient. Wherever they have an HIV patient, the responses are shameful"* (*Ibid.*). The situation of the PLWHA from this hilly region is made worse as they have to travel to NBMCH for medication, and especially if they are receiving ART, which are not provided at the district hospital Darjeeling.

One of the respondents said, *"Being a female and HIV positive makes my life difficult. When I go to the hospital the staff there looks at me with dismay. They think that I am a woman of bad character and this is the desired consequences of my behaviour. Though their reactions are not overt it can be felt how condescending they are towards us. They always seem irritated and shout whenever they have to deal with me in the hospital. They do not listen to what I have to say. They just throw the papers and are always in a hurry to get rid of me."* Such behaviour draws unnecessary attention towards these PLWHA as many have not disclosed their status to the public. As one of the respondents said, *"The constant shouting of some of the nurses draws unnecessary attention at me. As I have not disclosed my status publicly it becomes difficult for me to fight with the nurse and ask her to show some respect."* One of the respondents said, *"As Darjeeling is a small place generally everybody knows everybody. Somehow or the other people can know who a person is. We just want the health staff to be a little sensitive towards us and show us some respect but most of the time the nurse are shouting and ill-treating us. The news of our HIV status can become public if the health staff does not act in a responsible manner."*

As in the whole of the region there is only one hospital which looks after the PLWHA, there is no choice for them but to visit the Darjeeling district hospital. In case of those who are undergoing ART they have no choice but to access NBMCH. As there are just two agencies to choose from, the discriminatory response limits care and support for the PLWHA. When these PLWHA have to travel to NBMCH, their travel costs increases and as they are forced to travel longer distances, they perceived this to be unworthy. As one of the female respondents who is receiving ART from NBMCH said, *"We have no choice but to go to Siliguri for treatment. Given a choice I would never go there. There we face a lot of problems. The staff is never polite with us. We are always treated at the end when the doctor is in a hurry to go home. We have to waste the entire day for just five minutes with the doctor. The travel expenditure is also high. The nurses are worse than the doctors. They are constantly shouting at us. They think that they are doing us a service but they are actually always ridiculing us."* Another respondent who is also undergoing ART at NBMCH said, *"There is so much of discrimination there at NBMCH with regards to the people from the hills. They do not want to explain things in any other language other than Bengali. It is not a problem if they speak slowly and answer our queries but they do not want to entertain any questions we have. I wish there was an ART centre here in Darjeeling as well. It would solve so much of our problems. We can at least voice our needs here and there are doctors who support us as well. We spend the whole day standing on the queue and at the end of the day what we get is nothing but harsh words from the health staff. Apart from the doctors even the nurses and other staff misbehave with us. This is not what we deserve. The positive people's network in Siliguri also does not help us much in this regard."*

"We are facing problems in accessing Anti-Retroviral Therapy (ART) as we have to come all the way to North Bengal Medical College and Hospital for treatment and medication", said a member of Shanker Foundation, a network of HIV positive persons in Darjeeling town.[10]

Though the overall experiences of the PLWHA were not positive in the health setting, almost all the respondents had respect and admiration for a lady doctor in Darjeeling District Hospital. The respondents were thankful that they had her in the hospital. They felt that she understood their predicaments and helped them even if she was not on her duty. She had helped them in their quest for justice and had now and again told them about their rights and privileges. The most pivotal thing about her that was acknowledged by all was she was always patient with the PLWHA. One of the respondents said, *"She is such a nice person she is always supporting us. She calls us to find out if our health is good or not. She advises us not to indulge in things that are not beneficial for our health. She is always concerned about our well-being. She makes it a point to see that we are treated well in the hospital whenever we visit."* Another respondent said, *"Though I do not know much about her helping others but she has helped me tremendously. It is just because of her I am in here today. I wanted to die when I was told about my status. She counselled me and showed that I could live a life of happiness and fulfilment even with the virus. Today I go to her or call her up often and talk to her. There is so much of positive energy in her and this gives me a lot of desire to live and be optimistic in life. She has been a gift of God to me."*

PLWHA's Experience of Shanker Foundation

Shanker Foundation has been a boon for the PLWHA. All the PLWHA' experience of Shanker Foundation has been tremendously beneficial. They said that coming to Shanker Foundation's office has given them a new lease of life as they can meet people who are also going through the same ordeals in life and have similar experiences. They said that Shanker Foundation provides them a platform from where they can make their bitter life better by sharing their experiences and helping each other cope with the problems. They said that because of Shanker Foundation they have been able to find many friends even when they are infected by HIV/AIDS and when the whole world is isolating them. Because of Shanker Foundation they can avail medical facilities. The greatest experience of Shanker Foundation for the PLWHA has been the protection they perceive by being its member. They have gained respect from many sections of the civil society and say that the due must be given to Shanker Foundation. One of the respondents said, *"Had it not been for Shanker Foundation I would probably be dead by now. It is the courage given by Shanker Foundation that I am alive today. Seeing so many like me and sharing similar experiences has made me strong enough to tackle the negative impact of the infection. The bonding we have created helps us to live life and think beyond HIV/AIDS."* Another female respondent said, *"It is because of the members of Shanker Foundation that I am here in Glen Foundation. They take care of me and also my medical requirements. I do not have to bother much about anything. If it was not for the members of Shanker Foundation then how can a poor woman without a husband be able to live with such a fatal infection?"*

Shanker Foundation has been working for the welfare of the PLWHA. They have indeed been able to solve many of the problems faced by the PLWHA. One of the respondents said, *"The people[11] here in Shanker Foundation work overtime to provide all the help needed by the PLWHA. They take care of the travel if any of us have to go to Siliguri for any kind of medical help we require. They bring people from other places to help us feel positive. They take care of our nutritional needs as well by providing us financial support from other organizations. They do everything to make our lives better and happy."*

PLWHA's Personal Experiences

The PLWHA felt that their lives were no longer in their hands after they were diagnosed to be HIV positive. They were pessimistic about survival because they felt that HIV/AIDS was irreversible as they were aware that there is no medicine for its complete cure and as a consequence they anticipated death. One of the respondents said, *"Until a medicine or vaccine is developed or discovered we do not have any chance of getting well. I am speaking to you today but next time when you come I may not be alive. We are dependent on luck for survival."*

Earlier the PLWHA did not take it seriously whenever they fell ill, but now their perception and attitude towards illness has changed with time. Whenever they are ill now, their thought revolves around suffering and dying. They said that they are emotionally stressed out most of the time. One of the respondents said, *"Earlier I did not care a bit when I had fever or cough but now I just think that this could be the beginning of the end of my life. The thought of dying is such an agony that I cannot tell you how I live each day."*

Some of the respondents, married as well single had aspirations of raising a family but the disease has created doom and hopelessness as all of them know that regardless of the ART and other treatment available, there is no permanent cure for the infection. One married female respondent said, *"When I got married I thought of having babies, a daughter and a son, but when I was found to be positive all the dreams I had about life had to be buried. I gave up the idea of giving birth to a child. I was pregnant when I was diagnosed with HIV so I aborted the child. Though the thought of being a mother often comes and the desire is there I just cannot think of having a child. What would I do if the child is also positive? I cannot give suffering to an innocent child for my selfishness."* However, all the respondents were optimistic regarding the discovery of a vaccine that would cure their ailment. While, they were pretty sure that this would not happen in the immediate future and maybe not in their lifetime but they were happy that it would bring an end to the sufferings faced by their children. A widow said, *"Though there is no cure for HIV/AIDS now I am sure that the scientists will be able to find one soon. If they are able to find one it will at least solve the problems of the future generation, if not ours. I always pray to God to help us to find a solution to the problem of HIV/AIDS."* The thought that such a cure would not be available during their lifetime and being dependent on others during old age with the infection makes the PLWHA feel helpless. The prospect of the care giver abandoning them when they are old, weak and bedridden *'kills them'* as one of the respondents said. All the PLWHA were concerned about the attitude of the care givers and some said their parents were their care givers. However, this thought of troubling their old parents when they should have been taking care of them instead further destabilizes their life. One of the respondents said, *"I cannot imagine my old parents caring for me when I should be their support. It will not just be me but even my child who they have to look after. I wish I die before I have to see such days."*

PLWHA's Perception of the Community Members

The PLWHA feel that the community members have minimal knowledge about HIV/AIDS. They think that because of this factor they are discriminated. Though the PLWHA acknowledged the risk perception of the HIV sero negative people and their right to protect themselves from this fatal disease they think that their reaction is unwanted and much more than desired. One of the respondents said, *"Every individual has the right to protect oneself from any thing they think is dangerous to them. So if an individual protects herself/himself from HIV/AIDS I do not have any problem but the way they do it, is very humiliating. They should be able to think that we do not pose any danger to them and do not intend to harm them. They just react without having any knowledge about HIV/AIDS and this is very hurtful."* The PLWHA feel that the others think they are immoral people and so try not to have any contact and relationship with PLWHA. This attitude of the HIV sero negative people is due to the general belief that HIV/AIDS is transmitted by irresponsible sexual behaviour. One of the respondents said, *"They think we are immoral people and that our condition is the consequence of our misdeeds. They do not know that we are also like them and got the infection by accident."* PLWHA think that the community members do not want to know and learn about HIV/AIDS. They think that the community members live in a world of denial thinking that they cannot ever be infected by HIV.

The opinions of the PLWHA are influenced by the experience they have had with the others. They think that some of the health officials are not considerate about their situation and are therefore discriminatory in nature and attitude. They think that they need to spend more time with them and care for them sincerely. One of the female respondents said about the health officials, *"Even though they are the ones who should be protecting us they just treat you without any respect. Time and again they remind us how difficult our life is by ill treating and ignoring us. They just want to get over with us and do not spend much time with us. They are always in a hurry when they have to talk to us or conduct check up for any kind of health problem."* Another respondent said, *"Everybody here has somehow come to know that I am HIV positive and take undue interest in me. Though they are not directly involved in my treatment in the hospital they are always trying to eavesdrop when the doctor is with me. The doctor instead of asking them to leave just carries on and they end up hearing everything."*

The PLWHA perceive the politicians as their biggest 'enemies' as they have not done anything for them. Their plight has been compounded by the fact that the DGHC has not been functioning since 2002. This has made it difficult for them to receive help from the local government and this poses many financial problems. Due to the non-functioning of DGHC they are not receiving their grants on time and this creates a lot of problem in the functioning of Shanker Foundation, which invariably affects most of the PLWHA of Darjeeling hills. All the respondents were unanimous in saying that they have not yet received any help from the politicians. One of the respondents said, *"The politicians of this place are our biggest enemy. We see today there is so much of political will to fight HIV/AIDS, all around the world, but here in Darjeeling the politicians are just not there for us. They do not understand the issue and think that we are the concern of the health department and do not show any sensitivity. They say that the problem of HIV/AIDS can be solved in one stroke by getting all the people tested. Only if we had a strong political body then our fight to make ART available at the Eden hospital would have been easier."*

All the PLWHA perceived those people helping them to cope with the infection as godsend. They said that without these people their lives would have been very difficult. They said that without their help they would not have progressed so far as a network of positive people. They said that these people have helped them establish the Shanker Foundation and learn the official ways of doing things. They said that these people are real social workers and have helped them become triumphant over the stress and isolation they faced due to discrimination. All the volunteers who are helping the PLWHA are seen as true friends. One of the PLWHA said, *"With the help of these people we are here today. They provide us all sort of help financial, social, and emotional. They are always there for us and they respect our conditions. They treat us like one of them. They spend time with us everyday and this gives us immense self-belief and makes us think that we are also like any other human being."*

Though the experiences of the PLWHA were bitter, their reactions to the infectors were not negative. Though the PLWHA have gone through such ordeals it was found that they did not blame the person who infected them with this life taking virus but on the contrary it was found that they wished their life partners were still around with them and supporting them in these difficult times. The first hand account of the PLWHA and other respondents show that awareness regarding HIV/AIDS is abysmally low. Whatever little information they have is mired in wrong assumptions and prejudices. Extremely low levels of covert information regarding transmission and treatment of the virus coupled with almost non-existent medical facilities makes the hills a fertile ground for rapid spread of HIV/AIDS. For the PLWHA, the beacon of hope seems to be

Shanker Foundation, the sole positive people's network in the hills. But the researcher saw that the network still has a long way to go as far as any kind of sustained and fruitful advocacy is concerned. When compared to similar networks in India, Shanker Foundation lacks both in funds and in its capacity to politicize the issue and create a pressure in the administration to pursue their goals.

Notes and References

1. They are considered to be knowledgeable regarding HIV/AIDS and are therefore not included in the analysis of peoples awareness and knowledge about HIV/AIDS.
2. Bisexuals are people who have sex with both men and women but their predominant preference is men.
3. Decimal correct to two places.
4. Government services include all the people who have reported to be working in governmental offices. Some of the respondents said they were in services even though their salary suggests that they were casual workers.
5. Business includes all kinds of business as well as contractors. Includes FSWSs as well.
6. Includes those people who were not permanently employed by governmental offices, drivers and tea garden workers who worked when needed.
7. Those engaged in physical labour.
8. Includes Students and Home makers as well.
9. Kripa is a de-toxification centre at Darjeeling.
10. In an interactive session with the then Health Minister Mr. Ramadoss *(http://www.darjeelingtimes.com/news/News/India-not-ready-to-legalise-commercial-sex.html*
11. The office bearers of Shanker Foundation.

Chapter IV

Population Dynamics, Communication Technology and Vulnerability to HIV/AIDS in Darjeeling Hills

Every society is dynamic and in a state of constant flux, so the components of the society *vis-à-vis* the population is also dynamic. This state of flux is also brought about by economic developments and the desire to achieve a certain level of comfort in life. This chapter deals with mobility, sexual behaviour and trends among the people, risk groups, the knowledge and perception of HIV/AIDS among the people and also the stigma and discrimination associated with HIV/AIDS in Darjeeling hills.

Population Mobility and HIV/AIDS

The spread of HIV/AIDS in Darjeeling hills is roughly parallel with the rapid growth of Indian economy and globalization. Rapid economic growth, largely based on the Information Technology industries, brought about economic imbalances across the nation. During this period the attraction of job opportunities and the excitement and diversity of the cities attracted many migrants from Darjeeling towards the cities. Prior to economic globalization migration from Darjeeling was restricted to joining the armed forces, migration due to marriage, migration as domestic helpers and labourers. Migration from Darjeeling gained momentum when the employment opportunities there diminished drastically. Though lack of employment avenues is definitely a push factor there was also a pull factor as the new generation has become bolder and more competitive and sees things in a global perspective. Migration from Darjeeling is taking place for a large number of reasons. There are students migrating in search of better education facilities. There are people migrating for blue collar as well as white collar jobs. Migration in search of livelihood is conducive to the spread of HIV/AIDS as there is an absence of the institutions monitoring risk behaviour among the migrants and providing social support to them (Collins and Rau 2001). The freedom associated with being an independent working individual and the absence of parental restraints provides young workers with the opportunity to radically change their lifestyles. These lifestyles make them vulnerable to HIV/AIDS. Due to modernization and globalization rapid economic and social changes are taking place. These have provided the medium for behavioural changes that increases vulnerability to sexually transmitted diseases and HIV/AIDS. Migration increases the likelihood of infection due to ignorance of risk, lack of awareness and lack of access to health services.

Among the migrants, peer influence also plays a salient role in undertaking risk behaviour. This risk taking behaviour has been documented among a number of groups (Imem and Suwannarat 2002). Friends who have experienced drugs, alcohol and sex are also likely to induce others in their group. One of the respondents said, *"I had never had sex until I drank with a friend of mine. After drinking he asked me if I would like to have sex. When I said no, he insisted and just called a FSW and asked her to bring her friend along. I had sex for the first time."* When these migrants come home they form a bridge population for further transmission of HIV/AIDS and other STDs. The return of the migrants coincides with major festivals like Dusherra and Diwali when the use of alcohol is permitted even among the youth by the parents and is at its prime. Under the intoxicated state there is a likelihood of people engaging in risky behaviours and transmission of STI/STD and HIV/AIDS.

The residents of Darjeeling also frequently travel outside Darjeeling hills for short durations. They are likely to be exposed to infections. One of the respondents aged 27 said, *"I have travelled to a lot of places like Kolkata and Kathmandu and I have had sex there. Along with my friends I have had sex after drinking alcohol."* Another respondent, a driver by occupation said, *"Whenever I travel outside I visit brothels. If there is someone to accompany, then it is more exciting. Getting girls here in Darjeeling and Sikkim is very easy but a bit expensive. However in Siliguri it is cheap."* People generally want to experience sex in new places with new girls. As a respondent said, *"Going to different places and experiencing sex with different girls gives a different pleasure."*

The FSWs and the businessmen are one of the most mobile population. However, the businessmen are ignored as people tend to think that they are wealthy and form a small group and do not play any pivotal role in the dissemination of HIV/AIDS epidemic. What is not known is that they are exposed to sexual activities in all the places they visit. If they do not follow safe sex they can be a vector to all the FSWs whose services they avail as well as to their spouses. The businessmen are very much linked to the entertainment and sex industries. Their entertainment includes alcohol consumption and sex. Many of their deals are made over the drinking table (Sundas 2004). One of the respondents said, *"Our field is such that you have to keep your partner happy. His demands have to be fulfilled, be it alcohol or sex. Along with him you also end up drinking and having sex. Sometimes we are so drunk you do not know what you did the previous night."* Another respondent said, *"I am usually away from home for business. This is the time I get to have a lot of fun. Being a bachelor helps at such a time. You drink and have sex and I don't have to think about wife or kids. When I am away from home and alone my lifestyle is different."* Although they stay in other places for short periods only, this group is likely to bring STI/STD and HIV/AIDS to Darjeeling.

The FSWs are also a very mobile group. As there is no brothel based sex industry in Darjeeling hills their mobility is very difficult to track. They move frequently from one place to other for short periods of time. Now mobile phones have made their business a lot easier and they have become even more accessible to their clients. As one of the FSWs said, *"I am just a phone call away from my clients. Mobile phones have made it very easy to conduct business. Earlier we had to hang out at places but now we can stay at home and conduct business. Most of the clients these days ask for our number in case they require our services in the future. Our friends also have each others numbers so if there is any requirement we can just call each other. We don't have to stay in Siliguri, Gangtok or any place for days, the hotel people or our clients call us."* Most of the FSWs work throughout the district and also in neighbouring Sikkim. They say that they are very busy during the tourist season when business is at its peak. One of the FSWs said, *"Tourist season is very good for us. We can make a lot of money during this time of the year. During the tourist season both the locals as well the tourists use our services."* Some of the FSWs are not just confined to travelling across the district and Sikkim, they also travel to Delhi and Kolkata. Sometimes their travel expenditures are paid by the person with whom they are travelling. They say such travels are very relaxing and do not put any pressure on them as they are assured of their income. One of the FSW said, *"I like travelling with clients. All expenses are paid for and we have a lot of fun. You are not a FSW then. You don't need to worry about your daily income. But such travel is very few and far between."* One of the FSWs had at a point of time also worked in Delhi for two years. She said, *"Working in Delhi was such fun. We had taken up an apartment. The money was very good; we could earn thrice as much as what we earn here. Apart from working we did not have to fear any stigmatization. There our identities were concealed. People did not know what we did. There people were not bothered about us but here many know what we do for our living. The best thing about Delhi was we could wear the kinds of clothes we liked. I liked wearing half pants and t-shirts at home and could go out wearing them."*

The mobility of these FSWs is a big concern for the authorities. They may not know about their health status and may transmit the infection they are carrying to their clients.

Migration and health are intrinsically linked and a number of studies have provided ample evidence to support this. Migration is inevitably related with health problems, it is however not itself a risk factor. However, migration breaks down the social structures which are pertinent in generating conditions by which HIV/AIDS cannot spread easily. Migration especially under forced conditions, for example in conflict situation, or 'illegal' population movement, may lead to low status, low pay and/or isolated work and living conditions which increase vulnerability to a host of diseases. This is particularly true for women whose options are often limited to low status, low paid and/or isolated work like domestic helpers. Their low status and isolation from family and social support networks make them more vulnerable (Masanjala 2007).

People travel much more these days and 'are constantly engaging in significant sexual activities wherever they go at a time when AIDS is prevalent in society and in the process they spread the disease' (Mtika 2007). Nepalis migrate to work as domestic help and as labourers in the informal sector. There are agencies that recruit and bring them to Delhi. They become vulnerable to economic and social insecurities. Economic insecurities are manifested in the form of irregularity of employment, the casual nature of jobs, low payment and difficult working conditions. The migrants also face insecurities borne out of difficulties in the social domain like health hazards, alienation in the work place and isolation. These two insecurities are interrelated and they constitute a vicious cycle of insecurities for the migrants.

Nepali women who work as domestic helpers and labourers in other industries are exposed to both physical and sexual exploitation at the hands of the employers and the contractors. Being alone they look for companionship and intimacy. Their educational background and isolation acts as major barriers to information about STIs, HIV and AIDS and health services which renders them vulnerable (Sundas 2006).

A new trend of migration is visible among the people of Darjeeling. Recruiting agents are functioning in plenty in Darjeeling hills to take willing youth to foreign shores. Large numbers of youth are travelling to these places for jobs. The pay cheque is much higher. This gives them tremendous freedom as they do not have any familial restriction. Their only mode of enjoyment is drinking and having sex. One of the respondents who is working in Bahrain and had come for Dusherra said, *"It is fun there. We do not miss home as there are many of us from Darjeeling. We are given a flat and all of us stay together. Even the cook provided by the company is from Darjeeling. There is no shortage of recreational facilities. We have volleyball courts and football grounds but the best thing is beer is very cheap and girls from the whole of South and South-East Asia are available. What do you need more? Every holiday guys are out from morning till evening. It is cheaper for us to get the girls to our room than to take them outside. There is no dearth of beer in the room and we enjoy both beer and girl in the confines of our rooms."*

Another migrant said, *"I was there in Dubai for 5 years. I had the most exciting time of my life. Yes we had to work very hard but the rewards were worth it. The money was very good. Every weekend we used to organize parties and there used to be a lot of girls. Girls from India, Sri Lanka and from the South-East Asian countries used to come for the party. We had a lovely time. The girls also wanted to have fun and always looked forward to booze. After boozing most of the times we had sex. However, the Indian girls sometimes did not want to have sex and we had to convince them that if anything went wrong, like getting pregnant, then we would marry them. If this did not work then we would serve them more alcohol. Many of the guys who were staying together with their girlfriends never came for the parties. But most of the people going from here always joined the Dusherra celebrations. This was a big occasion. We used to get holidays for a week and there was a lot of drinking and if your luck favoured also a lot of sex."*

Boys and girls are paying a lot of money to go abroad for any kind of jobs. There are a growing number of females who go as domestic help to foreign countries. There is a possibility of such domestic helpers being sexually exploited. That many of them return home before the expiry of their contracts suggests that they must have been exploited. However, these domestic helpers give other reasons for coming back. One of the respondents aged 29 said, *"I missed my home and my kids very much so I wanted to come back. I knew before going that it would be tough but I had thought that I would be able to manage but once I reached there I could not stay. Though work was also not very tough but I could not stay."* Another married woman aged 30 said, *"I had gone to Hong Kong thinking that I will work for two to three years and earn some money. I had seen in movies that there the people do not do much work at home but once I reached there my employers got things that were kept in their store rooms for cleaning and washing. I thought this was it and continued for sometime. They started harassing me after a while. They started asking me to mop the floor twice a day. After working for 5 months I came back. It was like living in isolation. There was no one to talk and all day you were*

7alone and could not even handle the television properly. Some days the boss used to drink and create problems at home, he used to fight with his wife and break the plates and cups. This used to create more work for me. I could not stay in such an environment, so I decided to come home."

A young girl of 25 years who was working in Singapore at the time of the interview and had come home for vacation said, *"Working in foreign countries is very difficult. There are many issues which have to be tackled in a proper manner. You cannot leave the job after a few months after paying so much of money to the agent. Language is a major hurdle for anybody going to work in foreign countries. And at times there are things which happens which your conscience does not permit but you have to ignore such things. Comments are passed at you or during parties your employer's friends or even the employer tries to come very close to you after getting drunk or just touch you while passing. You are helpless at such times so it is always better if you ignore them."*

Joining the army is an age old tradition among the Nepalis. Official figures for people joining the army from Darjeeling hills are not available. It can be safely estimated that one-third of the migrants are those joining the armed forces. As studies conducted in the army suggest a considerable prevalence of HIV/AIDS among them, it can be safely inferred that those in the army from Darjeeling hills may also be infected by HIV/AIDS. The work environment and the pressure of being far away from home and family encourages these people to engage in risky behaviour. As they have to travel to many places in India and also abroad as peace keeping forces, it exposes them to a number of vulnerable situations. As one of the respondents has said that the lure and desire for new girl in a new setting is very difficult to resist. Job related stress and pressure also forces these people to engage in risky behaviour. Alcoholism is also a major source of risky behaviour. After drinking these people visit red light areas and use the services of the commercial sex workers. As one of the respondents said, *"In the army we are deprived of many things which we would like to have. We cannot take our family with us as most of the times we are moving from one place to another. This creates a lot of pressure on us as we are stressed and when we come back after doing the duty there is no one to talk to. Friends will also be out on duty and even if they are around the problem is not solved as they are also missing their families. This actually accentuates the problem. Under such circumstances, we just start to drink. While drinking if we think about our wives then we tend to go to the CSWs. If we had our wives with us then maybe we would not be visiting these places and women. Even the girls know that we are in need of sex that is why they are always near our barracks providing us services."* Another unmarried army person said, *"I am young and am not yet married. I would like to have as much fun as possible before I get married. I visit a lot of CSWs as nobody knows what I am doing. I need to gather experience before I get married. If I do not know the intricacies of sex then my wife may not be happy and may start having fun with other men when I am not at home."*

The tourists coming to Darjeeling are also a major threat to the spread of HIV/AIDS. There has been a sharp increase in sex tourism. Earlier it was only Darjeeling town that was the tourist destination but now other sub-divisions like Kalimpong and Kurseong have also been developed as tourist spots. Especially the tourists who are young and travelling alone are a threat to the propagation of HIV/AIDS. These young tourists come looking for sex. Even female tourists come looking for sex. As a waiter narrated, *"A lady was staying in our hotel for some days. I used to go to her room to provide the things she wanted like water, food etc. She was very nice to me and spoke politely with me. One night she asked for water and I as usual went to give her water. We started talking and all of a sudden she started touching me. After some time she took out some money and gave me. It was around 600 rupees and asked me to have sex with her. I had sex with her that night. It happened till the time she left the hotel and went. On leaving she gave me quite a lot of money as tips."* The nexus between the tourist, the hotel owners and the FSWs is also very evident in the hills. One of the FSWs, aged 30, said *"Tourists are the best customers. They do not bargain and there is no problem for payment. Our rates are told to them by the hotel owners. We go and visit them at the time given to us and provide them with the services. Older tourists are better as they pay you more and treat you well. They keep things quiet as they do not want anybody to know about their activity. They also give us more tips."* Another FSW said, *"There are many tourists who act in a weird manner. They want us to dance and sing as well. We are given extra money for these activities. They say they enjoy sex more when such activities are done."*

Condom use between the tourists and the FSWs is completely absent. One of the FSWs said, *"There is no condom use among us. Actually nobody talks about condoms. In fact when we are contacted by the hotel they ask us not to use condom."* The secretary of one of the NGOs in Kalimpong said, *"Here the influx of tourist is very high. They come here to have sex and there are so many FSWs available that they do not have any problem in fulfilling their objective. Though we are trying to make the FSWs aware of HIV/AIDS they do not take it seriously and do not ask their clients to use condoms. Tourists come here from many places and you do not know whether or not they have any infection. This makes the FSWs here and their clients susceptible to STI/STD and HIV/AIDS."* He further added, *"After working with these FSWs and some of their clients, there is supposedly an increase of condom use. However, the FSWs narrate that the clients are reluctant to use condoms as they say it reduces the pleasure of sex. Again the major problem regarding condom use in such paid sex is that the use of alcohol is very high and under its influence they do not use condom."*

Another important group of people in fanning the spread of HIV/AIDS are the IDUs. Though they are not as mobile as the FSWs their risky behaviour accompanying this restricted mobility is a threat. Generally, the IDUs move from one place to another in search of drugs. The IDUs in their desperation for a *'fix'*[1] do not mind fixing in the *den*[2] itself and do not care whether the needle they are using is sterilized or not. One IDU said, *"I go to Siliguri to get "maal"*[3] *and as soon as I get it I do it there itself. The desperation is such that I don't care to bother whether the needle has been used earlier or not. Generally, the needles there in the den are used by numerous people like me who come to get 'maal'. We generally go to Siliguri for 'maal' but if there are any news that someone from some place has got good stuff from some other place then we usually go to his place to get that stuff. We have to pay higher price when we get stuff this way. But such travel happens very less as nobody wants to sell the stuff they have got from far off places. We rely on Siliguri for 'maal' and only if we somehow have a lot of money then we travel to the North-East and to Kolkata. The trouble is worth taking as you can also sell the stuff at a higher price."*

Those in the government services are the ones who travel less. For them the unemployed youth gets the *''maal'.'* One IDU who is also a government employee said, *"There is no need for me to travel to get the stuff as the boys get it for me. I have to pay for their expenses and they do the job. They are doubly rewarded as they get to travel as well as get to 'fix.' They do not have to spend anything and at the same time they also keep some for their future need. However, I would like to go to Siliguri and buy the stuff myself. When I have time I go and buy it myself. I go to places where good quality 'maal' is available. I take a long leave and go to places like Manipur and Kolkata. There are friends in these places who help. We have great times together. We 'fix' together and show our bonding. Sex does not become important for me and I don't go looking for it and whenever I have had sex it is with fellow girls who also do drugs."* A female IDU said, *"I don't like to go to other places to get the stuff. Only when I desperately need it do I go to other places. Whenever I go to Siliguri they give me for lower price and offer me free fixes as well. However, they try to exploit me sexually as I am a girl."* A youth said, *"When we travel we do not carry the 'equipment'*[4] *individually as it is risky. We use the same 'equipment.' When we do the first fix we don't sterilize the needle. Only when we use it for the second time do we think of sterilizing it, that too many are not bothered."*

Sexual Behaviour and HIV/AIDS

The changes in the world around have had an effect on the socio-psychological behaviour among the youth in Darjeeling. The traditional values are fading at a rapid pace. Young girls are more willing to seek equality in every pursuit of life, including sexual pleasure, which was not considered important by their counterparts of the earlier generation. Due to modernization sex is no more a taboo. Premarital sex among the girls and boys has gained grounds. Much of the premarital sex is consensual and forced sexual liaison was not reported. There is a clear change in the attitude of young people towards virginity. According to a sociologist, *"There has been a definite change in the attitude to sex. Earlier when I spoke to girls about sex, they were embarrassed and perceived it as a taboo. Now they are more open and liberal at the attitudinal and behavioural level. Fewer urban bred, well-schooled girls condemn premarital and extramarital sex." (www.darjeelingtimes.com)*

Youth have become casual towards sex. Casual liaison, binge drinking and sex go hand in hand. One of the respondents aged 18 said, *"I was invited by my friend to his birthday party. Most of the guys and girls there were boyfriends and girlfriends. I was alone and was introduced to a girl who was also alone. We started to talk and after some time started to drink beer. We both got drunk. I don't know what happened and we started to kiss and after that we just had sex."* Due to the casual and experimental nature of sex these boys and girls are being exposed to multiple partners at a very tender age. They are not aware of the dangers of such sexual liaison. A 22 year old woman said, *"I feel sick every time I read one of the cover articles about all the diseases you can get from sex. I am just starting my life, I want to enjoy relationships. Someday I want to get married and have kids. It scares me to think that I could get some disease that will affect my body in the future, but that doesn't mean I am supposed to be suspicious of every new man I meet."* (*www.darjeelingtimes.com,* 2007). The eagerness to prove their masculinity among young men also introduce themselves to sexual activities (Mahalik 2007) which to an extent is also guided by the cultural demands of many societies. Respondents above the age of 40 generally thought that the sexual situation has changed drastically as compared to their times and that the sexual practices were more liberal among the younger people.

Multiple partners among the sample population is very much evident. Some had multiple partners before marriage but now were faithful to their wives. Some of the women reported having multiple partners because they were enticed by the attractive, expensive consumer goods that were available for exchange, revenge for a husband's infidelity or impotency. These factors are pertinent in driving women towards multiple partners (Tawfik and Watkins 2007). There are a high number of people reporting having multiple partners at a certain point of time. Among the male respondent's in the community members category there are 100 out of the 112 reporting having had sex with multiple partners. Out of the 42 females in the same category 25 reported having had multiple partners. Out of the 17 married women 9 reported having sex with multiple partners. Many of them said they had relations with multiple partners as their husbands were not at home and were outside their hometowns. This really poses a danger for the spread of HIV/AIDS. One married women aged 31 said, *"As my husband is not here I have had sex with a number of men in the past. He is still working in a foreign country and at times when there are moments of anxiousness and nervousness I call a friend, have some drink and just have sex. It makes me feel better."* Most studies on HIV/AIDS have only reported the danger posed by the husbands who go out in search of livelihood and indulge in risk behaviour but here a new trend is evident when the wives who were left behind at home are indulging in sex with multiple partners. All the bisexual also reports the existence of multiple partners among them. Among the IDUs as well, multiple partners is evident. A doctor of Darjeeling District Hospital said, *"The IDUs have multiple partners. They do not act responsibly as well. They have wives at home and have a fellow companion as their partner outside marriage. Even after counselling they don't try to understand that they are the most vulnerable and susceptible to HIV/AIDS. Most of the IDUs in Shanker Foundation who are married have infected their wives and may be many more outside marriage."*

Table 4.1: Sexual Behaviour of the Study Population

Type	*Premarital*	*Extra-marital*	*Sex with FSWs*	*Multiple partners*	*Sex while Travelling*
Male	98	36	74	100	74
Female	38	9	0	25	16
Total	136	45	74	125	90
Per cent	68.34	22.61	37.18	62.81	45.22

Source: Field Data.

From Table 4.1, it is evident that a large number of respondents were engaged in premarital and extra- marital sex. The percentage of both male and female indulging in premarital and extra-marital sex is high and accounts for 68.34 and 22.61 per cent respectively. 62.81 per cent have reported having multiple partners at the time of interview. Between the ages of 15 and 20 years there are rapid physical and emotional changes where parents cease to be the frame of reference and peer influence is at the utmost. At the same time, with the uninhibited lifestyles displayed on satellite television and in movies these adolescents indulge in youthful fantasies.

The number of people falling under this age group who have had sexual exposure was quite high. Out of the 30 in this age group 12 have reported having sexual experience. However, most of them have reported a single exposure to sexual experience. Most of them are buying sex in Siliguri. One of the respondents aged 19 said, *"I wanted to experience how it feels to have sex so when I was in Siliguri I went to Khalpara*[5] *and had sex there."*

Table 4.2: Respondents' Conversation about Sex

Gender	*Talk About Sex*	*With Friends*	*With Wife/ Husband*	*Talk About Wife/ Husband/ GF/BF*[6]	*Talk About Girls/ Boys*	*Talk About HIV/ AIDS*	*Talk About Condom Use*
Male	95	95	24	14/35	90	8	9
%	47.73	47.73	12.06	7.03/17.58	45.22	4.02	4.52
Female	45	45	5	18/20	18	5	3
%	22.61	22.61	2.51	9.04/10.05	9.04	2.51	1.50

Source: Field Data.

From Table 4.2, it is clear that a higher percentage (47.73%) of the male respondents speak about sex than the female respondents. The percentage of the respondents speaking about sex with their spouse is also higher for the male than the female. Though sex is still a taboo among the people but the influence of changing time is evident from the above table as people are speaking about it and importantly females are also willing to talk about sex.

There are a high percentage of male respondents who talk about girls they have had sex with their friends. All the respondents who have reported to have talked about sex have reported talking about it with their friends and 45.22 per cent of the male respondents have reported to speak about girls with whom they have had sex. There is a high per cent of single male respondents speaking about the last sexual act they had and whether or not they enjoyed it. Apart from this they also discuss the girl with whom they had sex with. This tendency among the males puts the identity of the girl in danger as the male discloses all the information of the girl and all share the phone numbers if the girl has given them. This act makes the girl vulnerable to coercion and blackmail from other boys as they may also want sexual favours from the girl. However, there is a lesser per cent of respondents who speak about their partners in sexual conversation. There are only 14 married respondents who speak about their wives when they talk about sex while there are only 35 single male respondents who speak about their girl friends. There is a high per cent of married female respondents who speak about their husbands while conversing about sex. 81.81 per cent among the married female respondents speak about their husbands while having conversation on sex. Their discussion about their husband revolves around the latter's promiscuity and infidelity. Only 9.04 per cent of the female respondents spoke about other boys while conversing about sex. There is a negligible per cent of both the male (4.02%) and female (2.51%) respondents who speak about HIV/AIDS while discussing sex and even fewer discuss condoms among the female (1.50) respondents. Condom is discussed only as a means to prevent pregnancy and not as a protection against STI/STD and HIV/AIDS. The 4.52 per cent of male respondents who discuss about condoms also saw it mainly as a means to prevent any kind of unwanted pregnancy. The low percentage of both the male and female respondents talking about their partners while speaking about sex with their friends reflects that sex among the partners is still considered a private affair.

Condom Use and HIV/AIDS

Condom is a proven barrier against HIV/AIDS. However, its use is not widespread among the people of Darjeeling. Young people significantly experience risky sexual activity within marriage and also in premarital sexual relationships. The absence of timely and suitable care and knowledge adversely affects their reproductive health outcomes including HIV/AIDS (Santhya *et al.* 2007). There are only 24 respondents who have reported using condoms in the sample. Among the community members only 21 respondents reported using condom, while none of the FSWs and the IDUs reported using condom. Out of the 9 bisexuals in the sample only 3 reported condom use (Table 4.3). Though people have multiple partners and are using the services of FSWs, the use of condom is minimal. Men are seen as making decisions regarding condom usage. One respondent aged 28 said, *"Only when my husband thinks that we need to take some precautions for the prevention against pregnancy does he use a condom. Otherwise we never use it."*

Table 4.3: Number of Respondents Reporting Condom Use

Category	*Male*	*Female*	*Total*
Community Members	19	2	21
IDUs	nil	nil	0
FSWs	–	nil	0
Bisexuals	3	–	3
Total	22	2	24

Source: Field Data.

Though the majority of women practice sexual fidelity within marriage the husband's irresponsible behaviour is a constant threat for them as they lack the decision-making power and cannot always insist men to use a condom. It becomes very difficult for the women to avoid taking risk within marriage and otherwise because they have less bargaining power (Panos 1990). Some women fear that if they insist upon condom use or even ask their partners to use a condom, they will endanger their relationship which gives them social status, emotional as well as financial support. Prevention and control of HIV/AIDS efforts still rely on the 3 concepts of 'Abstinence', 'Being Faithful' and 'Condom use'. Unfortunately, these concepts are not known to the majority of the people. Only 21 respondents were aware of this concept. Only 14 out of the 154 community members knew about it and among the IDUs, there was a comparatively higher per cent who did not know about this concept. Among the IDUs, there were only 4 male who knew about the ABC concept. None of the FSWs knew about this concept and among the bisexuals only 3 out of the 9 in the sample knew about the ABC concept (Table 4.4).

Table 4.4: The Respondents' Awareness about the ABC Concept

Category	*Male*	*Female*	*Total*
Community Members	10	4	14
IDUs	4	0	4
Bisexuals	3	....	3
FSWs	0	0	0
Total	17	4	21

Source: Field Data.

Females do not make decisions regarding condom use and therefore the rate reporting its use among them is low. One of the female respondents said, *"I don't know much about condom but sometimes I ask my husband to use so that I don't get pregnant but he does not listen and I have to do as he desires."* The use of condom among the married couples is very rare. The question of love, trust and faithfulness plays a salient role in the decision-making process. Condom may also symbolize extramarital relationship, sexual activity and so may be difficult to maintain or to introduce them into a long-term relationship. Issues associated with fidelity and trust of both male and female surface here (Manderson *et al.*, 2005). One of the respondents working with a national daily, *Telegraph* said, *"Though I understand the benefits of condom use I cannot talk to my wife about its advantages and make her understand. I cannot talk to her about condoms as she starts to question me on whether I trust her or not. She says she knows when she will and when she will not conceive. Though there are advertisements on television about condoms it is still beyond the comprehension of many girls and wives here. I think they are culturally conditioned to think that there should be no use of condom between a husband and a wife."* Another man of 28 years said, *"Why should I use a condom with my own wife, it is not needed. Condom only acts as a barrier to the trust and loyalty developed between a husband and a wife."*

Married women constitute a group with distinct risk of HIV/AIDS and face a host of obstacles in making informed decisions in protecting themselves from infections. Many studies conducted among HIV positive women conclude that considerable number of women were found to be infected only due to their exposure to sex with their spouse (NACO 2006).

The narratives of HIV positive women reiterate and substantiate the link of marriage and the risk of HIV infection. A PLWHA said, *"I was infected by my husband. He was a driver and used to come home late and at times he was away for days. He was ill once and even after days of treatment from the doctor at my place he was not recovering so we took him to Darjeeling District Hospital. After days of medication he was advised to get himself tested for HIV. He was found to be positive. I was also advised by the doctors to do the test. I also got myself tested. To my horror I was found to be positive. I felt like killing him for giving me this but what to do, he also may have not known that this would happen to him and so much of trouble would befall on the family."*

Another HIV sero positive woman said, *"My husband was married earlier and his wife was dead when he married me. I was pregnant and had gone for getting some tests done. I was told by the doctors to get HIV tested. They knew that my husband was positive so I was asked to do the test. I was found to be positive so I aborted the baby. Even my in-laws knew about their son's status and did not tell me about it. I wish he had been honest with me, I would not be living with this burden and by now would have had babies as well. I was just found to be positive in the month of March."* A nurse in Kurseong hospital said, *"Recently we had a case where a woman was brought with recurring fever and constant weight loss. So after initial treatment, when her condition did not improve, she was asked to get tested for HIV in Darjeeling. We found out that she was positive. We called her husband to learn about his wife's life history. It was found that he did not think that his wife could have got the infection from him. During the course of the investigation it was found that he had been living in Delhi for the past 4-5 years and had visited the red light area a number of times. We also asked her husband to get himself tested and he was also found to be positive."*

The premarital and extra-marital sexual experience of men and women are different. For the majority of women sexual activities mostly take place within marriage but most men (98) have experienced premarital and extra-marital sex. Condom use is also rare. Few women who have reported having premarital sex had sex with their regular partners on their insistence that they would marry them. While a majority of men have reported having sex with multiple partners and FSWs. Such behaviour suggests that men may already have a sexually transmitted infection or may be HIV positive which could have been transmitted to their wives or their partners.

There is a probability of HIV/AIDS transmission at a brisk rate in places and communities where there is a prevalence of multiple sexual partners, premarital and extra-marital sexual relations and the availability of prostitutes (Ford and Koetsawang 1991). In Darjeeling the presence of these factors and the absence of an effective health delivery system, provides a fertile ground for the rapid transmission of HIV/AIDS. The fact that significant proportion of young people are increasingly engaged in premarital sex indicates the erosion of traditional norms and values, which have acted as deterrent to deviant behaviour, considered risky for the spread of HIV/AIDS.

The closure of tea gardens, lack of employment opportunities, and the impact of modernization and globalization, and a high degree of consumerism, fostered by conspicuous opulence and lavish malls and departmental stores easily tempts girls to sell sex and make some extra income. The project officer of HSWS, Kalimpong said, *"It is very difficult to convince the FSWs to leave this occupation and take up an alternative profession as they are accustomed to a relatively high income."*

The pattern of condom use in Darjeeling cannot be ascertained because the records of condom sale are not maintained. The predominant sellers of condoms are the chemists and there are no condom vending machines. Conversation with the chemists brought out the fact that there are very few buyers of condoms and those few who come to buy still hesitate to ask for one. The socialization process and the cultural norms and values make sex a taboo. In such a situation people do not learn the advantages of condom use and consequently do not use them. Moreover, people's knowledge about condom is limited to it being a pregnancy control device. Female condom, which empowers women, is still unknown and many have not even heard about it. Women are also in a disadvantageous position as most of the sexual activities are initiated by the men and they possess no bargaining power, which renders them ineligible to negotiate on the use of condoms. Even the belief that condom use is associated with promiscuity impedes women from using it or asking their partners to use one.

Family Life Education and HIV/AIDS

In the hills there are no institutions providing family life education and the need for this was felt by most of the respondents. Among the male respondents 95 were in favour of family life education in schools while only 45 of the female respondents were in favour of it. Though the number of respondents in favour of family life education was high they were apprehensive about the negative impact it could have on the young school going children. As one of the respondents said, *"Sex (family life) education in schools is good but it has to be noted that things are changing very fast here. Young boys and girls are indulging in sex without having proper knowledge and if they are taught about it in school their curiosity might heighten and there will be more of them indulging in it. Even the culture and tradition has to be respected when we start to impart sex education in schools."* Guidance to the young pupil is the most important thing in the process of imparting family life education but this was a major problem and many of the respondents said that the absence of qualified teachers would have a negative impact on the students and lead them in the wrong direction.

The respondents who were against family life education were of the opinion that it would make it impossible to control the young generation. The impact of westernization and modernization was already felt by many and reported that young people were coming home late and in intoxicated states. They thought that if family life education was imparted in schools then the students would make wrong use of it. One of the respondents said, *"There is already so much of sex being heard about, among the school and college going people that if sex education is given to them then there will be more sex among the students as they want to know about what is being taught in school."*

Communication Technology and Spread of HIV/AIDS in Darjeeling Hills

India has witnessed a tremendous growth in communication technology. The reach of mobile phones has been unparalleled in the history of telecom industry. The world is coming closer due to the rise in the number of people using mobile phones and other technological advancement. Today everybody has become accessible and as a consequence the risk of HIV/AIDS spreading far and wide has also grown simultaneously. Today in Darjeeling almost everybody uses a mobile phone.

Darjeeling does not have a brothel based sex industry, so it was always a difficult proposition for those seeking the services of FSWs. Even the FSWs themselves had to encounter a lot of problems while seeking out their clients. Now that the mobile phones are in use the relational dynamics between the client and the service provider has changed dramatically. Today the relationship between a client and FSWs thrives on mobile phones and the contacts they make. Earlier when there were no mobile phones the FSWs had to wait for their clients at certain places but now they are available all the time because they could be contacted anytime. Their business hours have also increased significantly. Out of the 74 respondents who have reported using the services of FSWs, 69 have reported using their mobiles to avail the services of FSWs. All the 19 FSWs in the sample reported the use of mobile phones in conducting their business. All of them reported contact being made on their mobiles by their clients. A 25 year old FSW said, *"Two years earlier I always had to come to the town to look for my clients. Lot of time was wasted waiting for the clients but today I can go about performing any other chores and stay at home and at the same time am also connected with my clients. They can just call me if they want my services."* A 30 year old FSW vividly expressed the benefits that have been made by the advent of mobile phones in their business. She said, *"Today the girls who are in this business are lucky. They do not have to face the difficulty of finding clients as we did some years back. We used to stay in a hotel and look for clients. All the time we were concerned about others finding out about what we were doing. Today these girls just speak on the phone casually and without the knowledge of others around them while fixing appointments."* Another FSW said, *"Earlier we had to go to Siliguri and on occasions spent days without any work if our luck did not favour us but today we just rush to Siliguri when we get calls from the clients themselves or from the hotel. This way we save money as well as time."* Mobiles have also provided security to the FSWs. A 30 years old FSW said, *"As most of the business is done over the phone we can also ignore those clients who have not behaved properly with us. Earlier all the negotiations were done face to face with the clients so we could not avoid those with whom we were not comfortable. But today we can just make an excuse and avoid them or ask them to come to places where we are comfortable."* Another FSW said, *"The only problem we face and have to be careful about are the police raids but due to phones we are always alerted by our contacts."* The scope of their business has also expanded with the use of mobiles. 26 year old FSW said, *"Earlier not everybody used to come to us but nowadays as people don't have to speak directly with us many people are using our services. Well-to-do people as well as college students call us to find if we are available? Especially the respected people of the society want to maintain secrecy so they just give us the time and place on the phone and we go there."* Another 25 year old FSW said, *"Before we had mobile phones we were confined to a place but now we are more mobile. These days we get calls much in advance and also from far off places. This helps us fix everything accordingly. This way we do not lose out on time and business."* Mobiles have become the backbone of this business in Darjeeling hills. One FSW said, *"Today it would be impossible to do business without mobiles. Your business depends upon how much contact you have with your clients."*

It is not just the FSWs who are benefiting from the use of mobile phones but also those who seek their services. The clients are the ones who make the most of this technological advancement. One of the respondents said, *"Sex has become very easy these days in the hills. There are many who are into this business and mobiles have made it very easy to track them. If you have a number of one of them then you can use the services of the whole gang. If the one you call is not available then she herself makes arrangement for you as they would not want to lose out on the clients."* Another respondent said, *"If you have the contact number of a FSW then you can call her wherever you are."* Another respondent said, *"The use of mobile phones has made it very easy for the FSWs to work without any impediment. Earlier when they were working their reach was limited and they worked discretely. But today they are just a phone call away. Everybody seems to be happy and nobody is complaining."* One respondent who is married said, *"Mobile phones have made our life easy. Our work is such that you reach home late. You can be anywhere and with anybody and if you do not want your family members to know your whereabouts you just have to give a call and tell them that you are with your friends and at this place then they do not bother you. You can have fun."*

Mobile phones have also played a salient role in shaping the sexual role in other relations. As modernization has redefined the sexual orientation of the youth, mobile phones have played an important role. Mobile phones have become a status symbol so many young people want the best of the available phones. Those who cannot afford the best are selling themselves for it. There are both men and women who are taking advantage of this situation. A doctor in Darjeeling said, *"These days consumerism plays an important role in the kind of life you lead. Young people are engaging themselves in casual sex just to get the things they require. These days it seems that the item on the top of the list is mobile phones. There are many who would like to exploit this situation. They have lot of money and can afford to spend on sex. Even the girls are happy to provide services to this richer clientele as they are paid more and it is also safer as most of their clients have families and want to keep things as quiet as possible. They are in grave danger of being infected by HIV/AIDS, as they have multiple partners and their partners are not just confined to one place. However, we cannot do much to bring about changes in their lifestyles as they would like to hide their behaviour and project themselves differently."* Another respondent said, *"Speaking with your girlfriend for a long period develops an intimate relationship. It is not easy here to spend lot of time with your boyfriend or girlfriend. As you talk over the phone no one will bother you and a sense of intimacy develops between you and your girlfriend. Once this intimacy is developed there is no barrier to sex. Phones have brought all those in love very close and in touch for 24 hours."*

Alcohol Consumption and HIV/AIDS

Alcohol consumption among the people of Darjeeling is culturally prescribed. A very high percentage of the people in Darjeeling hills consume alcohol. The relation between alcohol consumption and health is very adverse in Darjeeling hills. This dire consequence is further accentuated when there is high risk sexual behaviour under the influence of alcohol. The nexus between substance abuse and spread of HIV/AIDS is now a well established fact. Substance abuse with its mood altering effect leads to deviant behaviour and lifestyles with greater possibilities of relations with multiple partners due to loss of self-control and unsafe sex.

The NIH Office of AIDS Research has identified alcohol use, abuse, and dependence as an important factor in the spread of HIV. Individuals who abuse alcohol are more likely to become infected and to infect others (*http://www.niaaa.nih.gov*).

People who use alcohol are more likely to engage in high risk behaviours like multiple partners and unprotected sex that places them at risk of contracting HIV/AIDS. Heavy drinkers are found to be more likely to have unsafe sex as defined by casual associations, non-use of condoms. In addition, there is a lesser likelihood of condom use among men who frequently combine alcohol and sex. Lower use of condom is also associated with young age and people (Manderson *et al*. 2005). Alcohol consumption no more remains the symbol of masculinity as there have been a growing number of women who also consume it. Earlier there were only older women drinking alcohol in the confines of their home but due to the changing times and profiles of the women, young girls are also drinking alcohol in bars and hotels. These places have become the hub of sexual activities as it is easier to find potential partners.

Alcohol consumption before sex is directly proportional to risky sex practices. The use of alcohol before sex has been reported by all the category of the sample population. The at risk group such as FSWs and bisexual have also reported alcohol use. The entire FSWs in the sample reported consuming alcohol with their clients. Almost 50 per cent of the bisexuals reported consuming alcohol before sex. 105 men among the community members have reported consuming alcohol before sex. Among the married women who have had extra-marital sex only 3 reported drinking alcohol before sex. The prevalence of alcohol consumption before sex among the respondents indicates that the existence of safe sexual practices is miniscule.

The sexual behaviour among those who drink before sex has been reported to be unprotected. One of the FSWs said, *"We are here to earn money and if our clients wants us to drink with them I do not have any problem with it. If we keep our clients happy they will also keep us happy."* Another FSW said, *"I do not know what I am doing when drunk."* Another respondent said, *"Alcohol consumption gives you a high and knocks you out of your senses. In such a situation you don't remember anything apart from having sex."* Further a respondent said, *"You spend so much money on the girls to enjoy so why would I use a condom and spoil the fun."*

A male respondent said, *"Drinking alcohol before sex gives me a sense of relief. There is no ill feeling of cheating on your wife. It diminishes all the inhibition of having sex with other people, and also gives me an excuse for this deviant behaviour."* Another respondent said, *"I drink to have sex. If I don't drink then I cannot have sex, it gives me that extra drive."*

Alcohol consumption among the FSWs is prevalent as they have to cope with the pressure of providing services to many clients. Adolescent youth are also consuming alcohol as they are hesitant about the casual sexual encounters. A 20 year old youth said, *"I had never experienced sex so to get over the fear I drank before having sex."* Sex and alcohol consumption is intrinsically linked in Darjeeling hills and as there are a large number of people involved in its consumption there is a constant threat of the spread of HIV/AIDS.

Flying Sex Workers and HIV/AIDS

As there is no brothel in Darjeeling hills it is very difficult to identify those who are engaged in this trade. Their identity remains hidden and it is difficult to make correct estimates about their numbers. This difficulty further arises as there are many who do not work on a regular basis. Their business is characterized by their mobility. Whether these FSWs work permanently or intermittently they are mobile and their reach is far and wide. Their mobility and reach is a great cause of concern for controlling and preventing the spread of HIV/AIDS.

The FSWs are very vulnerable to HIV/AIDS. The pace of transmission of HIV/AIDS involves a host of factors, but the most important issues are condom use, safe sex practices and the reproductive health of the FSWs and their clientele base. The generally held belief that condoms are a barrier to pleasurable sex also hinders many to use condom (Manderson *et al.* 2005; Nag 2001). The FSWs also have no or very little control over their clients and cannot force them to use condoms because they are powerless economically and otherwise. None of the FSWs in the sample reported having used a condom or having discussed HIV/AIDS with their clients. As the use of alcohol is also very much prevalent among the FSWs and their clients, any kind of inhibition regarding HIV/AIDS is also reduced under the intoxication of alcohol which also acts as an impediment to condom use. Further the presence of STD is a recognized co-factor in the transmission of HIV/AIDS and among the 19 FSWs there were 11 FSWs who had at certain point of time suffered from STD. Among the 154 respondents from the community members there were 36 who have reported to have suffered from some form of STD at certain interval of time. Out of these 36 respondents there were 12 females and 24 males who have reported to have suffered from some form of STD. Among the 9 bisexuals there were 4 respondents who have reported to have suffered from some form of STD at a certain point of time. Among the 17 IDUs in the sample there were 5 who have reported to have suffered from STD. Excluding the PLWHA there were 56 respondents who reported to have suffered from some form of STD and this translate into 28.14 per cent. This indicates that the FSWs and the other sub-groups do not have safe sex and regular medical check-ups. Their ill-health will further facilitate the spread and transmission of HIV/AIDS.

The FSWs in Darjeeling hills cater to the majority of local clients. However, there is a broad clientele base for the FSWs even among the tourists. As Darjeeling is a tourist destination, there is a large influx of both domestic and international tourists. It is, therefore, highly possible that both of them may infect each other if positive, and subsequently their respective families and clients. The high mobility of both the local clients and the FSWs themselves may transmit the virus to others and thereby create a vicious cycle. In particular, whereby the FSWs and their clients keep close relations with their homes and villages there is a potential for accelerating the spread of HIV/AIDS to newer places and population.

Intravenous Drug Users and HIV/AIDS

Among the intravenous drug users, HIV infection is transmitted primarily through contaminated injecting equipment, specifically needles and syringes. Drug paraphernalia is frequently shared by one or more individuals at the time drugs are injected. Those who may or may not themselves be IDUs but are sexual partners or wives of HIV infected IDUs are also at the risk of HIV/AIDS infection from them (Rhodes and Malotte 1996).

The first case of HIV in Darjeeling was found among the IDUs. Except for the Red Cross and the Kripa Foundation there are no agencies which have any records about the IDUs. These organizations are only able to document the records of those IDUs who come there for registering for NSEP or OST and rehabilitation. The availability and accessibility of drugs has been a major factor for the increase in the number of drug users in Darjeeling. Drug use is not tolerated in the hills. However, the prescribed socio-cultural use of alcohol is also responsible for fostering a large number of youth into drugs. Historically, drugs and injecting drugs was unknown to the people of Darjeeling hills. With the rise in socio-economic condition of the people during the late 1980s and early 1990s, corresponding with the Gorkhaland agitation, the use of drugs also grew in Darjeeling hills.

Post-Gorkhaland agitation has seen a significant rise in the smuggling of drugs into Darjeeling hills from the plains and the north-eastern states. Both the consumption and selling of drugs can be attributed to unemployment. As employment generation has been negligible most drug addicts have themselves has taken up this job to supplement their expenditure. Also high unemployment rates have led to increased levels of frustration among the educated and qualified youth. As a consequence many are taking drugs. Among the 17 IDUs in the sample, there are 13 who have completed bachelor degree and 1 who has completed master degree.

Drug addiction has a social aspect to it, it is seldom done alone. The IDUs inject in the presence of their friends. They are also initiated into it under peer pressure. The rapid increase in the rate of HIV transmission among the IDUs is because of the sharing of needles and syringes amongst them (Ford and Koetsawang 1991) in Darjeeling. The entire sample has reported sharing needles with their friends at the time of doing drugs.

There is a greater societal concern of HIV/AIDS being transmitted via the FSWs. The combination of these two groups is very potent for the spread of HIV/AIDS. Both these sub-groups have risky behaviours. The disinhibiting effect of some drugs results for many IDUs in increased sexual desires and enjoyment and may cause them to engage in unprotected sexual acts (Rhodes and Malotte 1996). The IDUs in the sample have reported using the services of FSWs and the presence of multiple partners in their life. All the IDUs in the sample have reported having sex without using condoms and all the male IDUs have reported having sex with FSWs and commercial sex workers outside their place of residence. As one of the female doctor of Darjeeling District Hospital said, *"Most of the IDUs have sex partners and they act very irresponsibly even though they are inducted in awareness programmes. When they are not intoxicated they are good but when they are intoxicated or need the money to buy drugs they act in an irresponsible manner. The female IDUs do not mind selling sex to do drugs."* A practice common among women, is to finance their crack habit by routinely exchanging sex for drugs with multiple partners, usually without using condoms (*Ibid.*). The IDUs have also reported to have shared needles with other drug addicts and had sex with the commercial sex workers when they have gone out to Siliguri or other places to buy drugs. This poses a greater threat for the IDUs of the hills as needle sharing is a common feature among them. As many of the IDUs are married they pose a greater danger to their family being infected by HIV/AIDS. The IDUs also consider themselves to be useless and so do not come for treatment and just carry on with their lifestyles. As the same doctor said, *"These IDUs do not consider themselves to be useful and insist on leading their lifestyles and do not come for any help. They think their life is over as they are found to be positive. One person, who was a drug addict, was found to be HIV sero positive. Even after counselling he did not think his life was worth living and carried on with his behaviour. Finally he died of overdose."*

Bisexuals and HIV/AIDS

The risk of becoming infected with HIV increases in direct proportion to the number of receptive and anal intercourse partners and men who reduce such practice significantly also reduce the chances of getting HIV infection (Kingsley *et al.* 1987). This sub-group is the most difficult to locate among all the other sub-groups as their number is less in comparison to the other sub-groups. Due to cultural practices people look down upon them. As a consequence they are hidden and do not want to disclose their identity. They are also a very vulnerable group as they do not want to mix with others and are confined within their groups. One bisexual said, *"I had to drop out of school because of peer pressure. Though there is a drop-in centre for people like me, people jeer at us when they see us gathering there."* The isolation of the bisexuals acquire greater poignancy in the context of HIV/AIDS. Their plight is further intensified by the Section 377 of the Indian Penal Code which states, "Whosoever has casual intercourse voluntarily against the order of the nature with man, woman, or animal shall be punished with imprisonment for life, of imprisonment for a term which may extend to 10 years, and shall be liable to fine."

Among the 9 bisexuals 4 have reported to have suffered from STD and got treated outside of Darjeeling. Within them they have multiple partners and the prevalence of alcohol use while having sex is very high. This sub-group is restrained from practicing safe sex in general and using condom in particular because of alcohol and drugs abuse among such populations (Wanigaratne *et al.* 2005). All the 9 bisexuals in the sample have reported having had sex with multiple partners. The use of services of FSWs is also very high. 8 of them have reported using the services of FSWs. They not only use the services of FSWs but also serve other bisexuals and MSM. They go to Siliguri to serve those who need their services. Their sexual orientation puts them at a higher risk of being infected by HIV/AIDS. As 4 of the bisexuals in the sample are married they can infect their wives at home. An official of Manas Bangla, Darjeeling said, *"It is very difficult to bring them into our fold as they are few in number and do not want to disclose their identity. They are the most at-risk group here as they are not aware of the dangers of unprotected sex and do not seek treatment when they are affected by STDs. Not only these they have multiple partners, they use the services of FSWs and also provide services to clients. They do not want to come out in the open even after being counselled by peer educators."* Another official of Manas Bangla said, *"There is a high incidence of STIs among the bisexuals in Darjeeling as they are not open to the use of condoms and lubricants. Every month we receive 5-6 cases of STI among them though there are very few who visit us. Even after telling them about the advantages of condoms and lubricants they are reluctant to use them."* The former official further said, *"As the number of MSM infected with HIV/AIDS, in the whole of West Bengal is the highest in Siliguri those who go there for sex is in greater danger of being infected by HIV/AIDS. If they get infected there they may in turn infect others here."*

Knowledge and Perception of HIV/AIDS among the People of Darjeeling Hills

Having heard about HIV/AIDS does not necessarily reflect the person's knowledge about the infection or the virus. Most people know that HIV/AIDS can be transmitted from one human being to another. However, they lack in precise understanding of how this transmission takes place. Even myth and misunderstanding surrounds the modes of transmission of the virus (Ramasubban and Rishyasring 2005). All the respondents in the sample have reported to have heard about HIV/AIDS from some source. However, their knowledge about it can at the best be said to be poor and confusing. Among the 199 respondents (excluding the PLWHA) only 12 respondents knew all the 4 modes of HIV/AIDS transmission and they all belonged to the community members' sub-group. 32.66 per cent of respondents knew about three modes of transmission and 8.54 per cent did not know any mode of transmission of HIV/AIDS (Table 4.5). None of the FSWs, the IDUs and the bisexuals knew all the 4 modes of transmission. There were 13 respondents who have reported other mode of transmission such as kissing.

From Table 4.5, above it is clear that the number of respondents who knew all the 4 primary modes of transmission is very less and comprises only 6.03 per cent and those knowing

Table 4.5: Showing the Respondents' Knowledge of Modes of Transmissions[7]

Type	*All 4 Modes*		*At least 3 modes*		*At least 2 modes*		*At least 1 mode*		*Don't Know*		*Total*
	M	*F*	*M*	*F*	*M*	*F*	*M*	*F*	*M*	*F*	
Community Members	8	4	33	4	27	7	31	25	13	2	154
FSWs	0	0	0	3	0	4	0	11	0	1	19
IDUs	0	0	14	3	0	0	0	0	0	0	17
Bisexuals	0	0	8	0	0	0	0	0	1	0	9
Total	8	4	55	10	27	11	31	36	14	3	199
Percentage	4.02	2.01	27.64	5.02	13.57	5.53	15.58	18.09	7.03	1.51	100.0

Source: Field Data.

only three modes of transmission comprises of 32.66 per cent. The corresponding figure for those who know only two or one mode of transmission is 19.09 per cent and 33.66 per cent respectively. Sex was the known primary mode of transmission for those who reported to have known only one mode of HIV/AIDS transmission. Those who did not know any of the primary modes of transmission are 8.53 per cent. Table 4.5 suggests that the women are less aware than men with regards to the knowledge of all modes of transmission. However, the number of female respondents who know only one mode of transmission is higher than the male respondents. Although the number of respondents associating HIV/AIDS with sexual activity is very high, the prevalence of premarital and extra-marital sex among the respondents, the absence of condom use and the utilization of FSW's services for gratifying their sexual desires makes them very vulnerable and susceptible to HIV/AIDS. Moreover, the percentage of men who did not know any route of transmission of the virus is higher than the women and this is an issue of concern as they are the ones who are primarily engaged in risk behaviours. These factors make the whole region very conducive for the spread of HIV/AIDS.

VCCTC is the backbone for the control and prevention of HIV/AIDS. They also provide other services like counselling to all the people who would like to know about HIV/AIDS and would also like to get themselves tested. However, very few people knew about the presence of VCCTC in Darjeeling District Hospital. Only 31.65 per cent of respondents barring the PLWHA, had heard about the VCCTC. 68.33 per cent of respondents did not know about the VCCTC being there in the district. However, the percentage of the respondents having visited the VCCTC was very low at 5.01. Among all the 199 respondents (excluding the PLWHA) only 3 female respondents had ever visited the VCCTC (Table 4.6)

VCCTC which is a salient feature of HIV/AIDS control and prevention is known to very less number of respondents. The number of respondents who have heard about VCCTC is very small as compared to those who have not heard about it. The number of female respondents among them is even less. Among the respondents who reported having heard about the VCCTC none were able to say since when the VCCTC had been

Table 4.6: Number of Respondents Who Know About VCCTC

Type	*Heard About VCCTC*		*Know About VCCTC in the District*		*Not heard about VCCTC*		*Have Visited VCCTC*	
	Male	*Female*	*Male*	*Female*	*Male*	*Female*	*Male*	*Female*
Community Members	37	10	37	10	75	32	1	2
FSWs	0	6	0	6	0	13	0	0
IDUs	6	1	6	1	8	2	5	1
Bisexuals	3	0	3	0	6	0	1	0
Total	46	17	46	17	89	47	7	3
Percentage	23.11	8.54	23.11	8.54	44.72	23.61	3.51	1.50

Source: Field Data.

functional in the district. Only 14 respondents among the 49 interviewed in Darjeeling reported having heard about VCCTC and its presence in the district although the VCCTC is situated in Darjeeling town itself. Among the 199 respondents only 10 have reported ever visiting the VCCTC and among them 3 are females. None of the FSWs have ever visited the VCCTC which shows their lack of awareness and also their unwillingness to use the services of the VCCTC. Only one among the bisexuals has reported ever visiting the VCCTC. The lack of knowledge of the VCCTC among the community members as well as the high risk groups threatens Darjeeling hills with the spread of HIV/AIDS.

The awareness regarding the prevention of HIV/AIDS among the people is even lower compared than the knowledge of HIV/AIDS itself. Most of the people have not heard about the concept of 'ABC', which is fundamental to the prevention of HIV/AIDS. This concept has been accepted the world over to fight the further spread of HIV/AIDS epidemic. However, the knowledge about it is absent among the respondents and only 21 respondents have reported to have heard about it. However, they did not know what it meant. Some thought the abbreviation, meant *"Always Be Careful."*

The people of Darjeeling hills think that HIV/AIDS is not related with the socio-economic or the political condition of the area and that it is completely a medical problem. The number of respondents who said that HIV/AIDS was a medical issue was an overwhelming 134 and comprised of 67.33 per cent of the sample. The majority among the vulnerable sub-groups also said that HIV/AIDS was a medical issue. Among the FSWs 10 out of the 19 said it was a medical issue while the corresponding figure for the IDUs and the bisexuals were 11 and 9 respectively. 100 per cent of the bisexuals said HIV/AIDS was a medical issue while 64.70 per cent of the IDUs reported it to be a medical issue. 19.09 per cent among the 199 respondents reported being confused whether HIV/AIDS is a medical or socio-economic issue.

Table 4.7: Respondents' Views about HIV/AIDS as Medical or Socio-Economic Issue[8]

Type	*Medical*	*Both M and SE**	*Don't Know*	*Total*	*% Medical*	*% Both*	*% Being Confused*
Community members	104	24	26	154	52.26	12.06	13.06
FSWs	10	2	7	19	5.02	1.01	3.51
IDUs	11	1	5	17	5.52	0.50	2.51
Bisexuals	9	0	0	9	4.52	0	0
Total	134	27	38	199	67.33	13.56	19.09

Source: Field Data.

The respondents were unanimous in declaring that the health infrastructure was not sufficient enough to control the infection and there is a need for more trained and compassionate doctors in the hospitals of the three sub-divisions. A male respondent, age 24, from Kurseong said, "*For most of the illness we are immediately referred to the NBMCH and most of the time there is no medicine or staff in the hospital. So how can these people provide care to those infected by HIV/AIDS?*"

Only 11 respondents have reported that the health infrastructure is developed enough to tackle HIV/AIDS in Darjeeling. The respondents were also of the opinion that there were not enough trained doctors for the control of HIV/AIDS. 177 respondents knew that HIV/AIDS was not a curable disease and 12 reported not to have known whether it was curable or not. The number of respondents reporting that there was medicine to control the progress of HIV to AIDS in a person was only 17 among the 199 respondents.

The females generally lacked knowledge about HIV/AIDS and safe sex. Cultural practices and beliefs have also acted as an impediment for them to garner knowledge about sexual practices and HIV/AIDS. As 192 respondents have reported sexual intercourse to be one of the modes of transmission it becomes imperative for them to understand and know about safe sex as the majority of the respondents do not use condoms while having sex. The knowledge of the concept of ABC which is the foundation for the prevention of HIV/AIDS is also very limited among the respondents. Among the respondents excluding the PLWHA only 21 have reported to have heard about the concept. The lack of knowledge of condom use and the concept of ABC has a direct implication on HIV/AIDS and also on women. It is very much essential that they are made aware of these things.

Those who lack awareness as well as those who are aware of the risk of unprotected sex, do not always perceive themselves to be at risk to HIV/AIDS. There are only 76 respondents among the community members who perceive themselves to be vulnerable to HIV/AIDS. Among the 19 FSWs, 18 of them have reported to being vulnerable to HIV/AIDS. Though the rate of those reporting vulnerability to HIV/AIDS among the FSWs is high, they do not have the knowledge to protect themselves from it. The general lack of awareness among them will also have an impact of HIV/AIDS transmission among the population.

Even among the health care staff the knowledge about HIV/AIDS were found to be incorrect or incomplete. It is of concern that 2 among the 8 health care staff were not aware that HIV could be transmitted through breast feeding. In the rural areas the health care staff requires more training regarding the ways by which HIV can be transmitted.

Most respondents perceive HIV/AIDS to be a major problem of life. Many say that it would ultimately bring death to the person suffering from it. Relating HIV/AIDS to death many thought that it was better to live a fun filled life than to die without enjoying the many pleasures it has to offer. Such hedonistic attitudes will further add fuel to fire.

Stigma and Discrimination in Darjeeling Hills

Though there is no literature on discrimination, stigma and denial in Darjeeling, there are evidences that these aspects of HIV/AIDS are very much prevalent in the hills as well. All the PLWHA in the sample have testified to being discriminated at certain point of time. Since they have not disclosed their positive status they report facing minimum discrimination at the hands of the community members. However, they report discrimination in the hospital settings. They report being ill treated by the nursing staff and who look offended when PLWHA visit the hospital. One female PLWHA said, *"Going to the hospital is a problem for me. The nurses there shout without reasons and try to stay as far away as possible from me. Her constant shouting draws unnecessary attention. She does not realize that her act may disclose my status to the others around. At times they don't even give medicine in my hand."* Another PLWHA said, *"These nurses and doctors are said to be second only to God but if you see the way they behave with us you will start to hate them. Especially the nurses are very rude to us. Last time I had gone to the hospital as a new entrant here in Shanker Foundation are required to do some tests. She just did not want me to touch her. I was just trying to tell her that touching does not transfer the virus she complained that I misbehaved with her."*

Discrimination is also reported at the familial and the community level though the degree is not very high. Those facing discrimination at these levels are women, as is evident in the rest of the country. A male doctor of Kalimpong Sub-Divisional Hospital said, *"Incidences of discrimination is evident here. In Lava village a girl was chased out of the home by her in-laws. The husband died of HIV/AIDS and she was blamed for transmitting the virus to the husband. The husband was actually working in Mumbai and was infected there. The in-laws now say that their daughter in-law has gone to her natal home and is not returning on her own and they have nothing to do with it. However, it was the in-laws who have chased her away as the villagers were witness to the whole incidence."* A PLWHA staying in Glen Foundation, Kalimpong said, *"After my husband died I was also diagnosed to be HIV sero positive. When my family came to know about it they stopped talking with me. I was isolated within the family. My condition was deteriorating and I was very ill when my Chema Sashu*[9] *came to my rescue. She along with her husband took me to their place. They took care of me but it became economically very difficult for them, as I had to take ARVs soon after. I was brought here with the help of members of Shanker Foundation. They come to visit me even though they are far away but no one from my own family visits me, not even my kids."*

The fact that most of the PLWHA in Darjeeling have not disclosed their positive status to their family also suggests that there may be some form of discrimination within the family and outside the family. A PLWHA said, *"I do not want to disclose my positive status to my family as they will be ashamed of me and my behaviour. Though I am sure my mother will understand it I am not sure about my father. What will I do if they ask me to leave the house?"* They also do not want to disclose their status as they fear stigmatization and rejection. This fear also contributes indirectly to their isolation.

In the employment sector as well there have been reports of discrimination. The local daily *Himalaya Darpan* dated 25th November, 2006 reported how a person was debarred from getting a job in place of his mother as he was HIV positive. The person was found to be positive when the sample of the blood donated by him was tested. This also highlights the fact that the issue of confidentiality is not taken care of by the health officials.

Discrimination against the person infected by HIV/AIDS is also rooted in the low level of awareness and knowledge of the disease. A respondent said, *"It is always good to keep a positive person away from the community as the disease is very contagious like T.B. and can spread very fast if they are allowed to stay within the community."* Only 14.07 per cent of the male respondents wanted to sit with a PLWHA.

The lowest discriminating tendency is evident among the high risk groups of the IDUs (64.70%), followed by the bisexuals (44.44%) and the FSWs (36.84 %). This tendency among the community members is mere 12.33 per cent (Table 4.8). This high degree of acceptance shown by the high risk groups can be due to the fact that their friends and colleagues might have been infected by HIV/AIDS and they themselves might think that they are also vulnerable due to their high risk behaviour.

Table 4.8: Discriminating Attitude Towards PLWHA

Type	*Sit with PLWHA*		*Allow PLWHA in Community*		*Allow +ve Children in School*		*Allow +ve teacher teach*		*Touch PLWHA*		*Care PLWHA*		*Percentage of individual Sub-Group*
	M	*F*	*M*	*F*	*M*	*F*	*M*	*F*	*M*	*F*	*M*	*F*	
Community members	16	3	16	3	16	3	16	3	16	3	16	3	12.33
FSWs	0	7	0	7	0	7	0	7	0	7	0	7	36.84
IDUs	8	3	8	3	8	3	8	3	8	3	8	3	64.70
Bisexuals	4	0	4	0	4	0	4	0	4	0	4	0	44.44
Total	28	13	28	13	28	13	28	13	28	13	28	13	

Source: Field Data.

The percentage of respondents who wanted to care for the PLWHA is 14.03. There were 22 respondents among the community members, 9 among the FSWs, 13 among the IDUs and 4 among the bisexuals who wanted to care for a PLWHA and comprised of 24.12 per cent. There were as many as 127 among the community members, 9 among the FSWs, 6 among the IDUs and 4 among the bisexuals who thought that restricting the movement of the positive people was necessary so that they would not infect others. The high number of IDUs willing to care for those suffering from HIV/AIDS may be because of the fact that they are aware that they are vulnerable and that many of the PLWHA at present are erstwhile IDUs.

Stigma and discrimination towards PLWHA may result in individuals denying they are HIV-positive and becoming less engaged in preventive behaviours and less likely to seek medical treatment. When sufferers attempt to receive medical treatment, they may experience a lack of commitment and even mistreatment by health professionals. Social segregation, increase in emotional anguish and loss of social support and network among the PLWHA are few important consequences of sigma and discrimination (FHI 2004). Stigma and discrimination may also deter individuals from seeking voluntarily testing for their HIV status.

The situation in the hills is ripe for the spread of HIV/AIDS in an emphatic way. The risk behaviour among the risk groups and among the population indicate that HIV/AIDS can spread in the hills like wild fire. The level of understanding and awareness regarding HIV/AIDS among all the people of the hills is negligible and this can be fatal for the people of this area in confronting the disease. There is a lot of work required for generating awareness among the people and the work which has been done with regard to the epidemic by the different governmental institutions, NGOs, families and community in Darjeeling hills will be discussed in the next chapter.

Notes and References

1. *Fix* is the term used for injecting.
2. *Den* is the place where they get the stuff, brown sugar and also the place where they usually do the fixing.

3. *maal'* refers to the brown sugar; also the word stuff is used. '*Saman*' is the word they use which has been translated into stuff.
4. Equipment is the word used for the syringe and the needle.
5. Khalpara is the locality in Siliguri where the brothel is located.
6. GF means Girl Friend, BF means Boy Friend in the local conversation.
7. Here in the table PLWHA are not included as all of them knew the modes of transmission as it was also taken for granted that they would know it even if they did not know before being infected by HIV.
8. PLWHA are not included in this
   * M= Medical, SE= Socio Economic
9. Chema Sahu is the younger sister of mother-in-law.

Chapter V

Response to HIV/AIDS in the Hills of Darjeeling—From Global to Regional Institutions

HIV/AIDS is a humanitarian as well as a health crisis. After the first case of HIV/AIDS in India was detected in Chennai, two decades ago among the sex workers, the epidemic has grown unprecedentedly. This growth of HIV has brought into action a multiplicity of actors for its control and prevention. A lot of targeted interventions programmes have been implemented. The responses have been rich in diversity and actors ranging from international institutions to local NGOs have played their role. Even then the citizens of India are not well-versed with the tools and techniques of confronting the challenges posed by HIV/AIDS. This is due to the lack of access people have to coherent sources of HIV/AIDS information (Ramasubban and Rashyasringa 2005).

People still believe that they are immune to HIV/AIDS as they are not involved in risk behaviours and that it can only affect those who are immoral and deviant. Today the international, national and the local NGOs as well as other civil society groups in collaboration with the government are working towards acquainting the citizens with the complexity involved in controlling and preventing the progress of the epidemic. As intervention and prevention programmes involve sensitive issues like sexual behaviours (which still is a taboo subject), and drug abuse (which is considered an unacceptable deviant behaviour), the NGOs working at the local community level are at a vantage point when compared to the international NGOs (who have more funds and technical expertise) and government agencies. Government institutions cannot work as effectively as the local NGOs, as commercial sex and drug abuse is a criminal offence and those involved in such activities do not trust the government personnel. This chapter gives a brief account of the international responses to HIV/AIDS and also sheds light on the responses from various institutions in the hills of Darjeeling, to control and prevent the epidemic.

International Responses to HIV/AIDS

HIV/AIDS is now being recognized not merely as a medical problem, but a social and developmental problem by the global community. Every year the number of people infected by the disease is increasing and as a corollary to this the number of people affected is also increasing.

However, UNAIDS 2007, the report on the global scenario of the epidemic for the first time reported that the number of those infected have decreased due to the rigorous exercise undertaken to access the intensity of the epidemic in India. This exercise resulted in calculating the number of PLWHA in India which was found to be lower than previously reported. This along with the fact that some of the estimates of the sub Saharan countries were also revised led to the overall reduction in the number of PLWHA globally (UNAIDS 2007). However, people have argued that there were flaws in the methodology applied in approximating the number of PLWHAs (Bagla 2007). The 2010 global HIV/AIDS update published by UNAIDS reports that globally there are 33.3 million adults and children living with HIV/AIDS and worldwide the number of infection has gone down by 19 per cent (UNAIDS 2010).

Under these circumstances a firefighting response and the involvement of the civil society is urgently required to prevent the further spread of the epidemic as it was affecting the poor and the marginalized segment of the population. At the same time the costs of essential drugs are also beyond the reach of the poor and policies such as 'structural adjustment programmes' further accentuated the plight of those infected and affected. The Medecins Sans Frontiers expressed concern

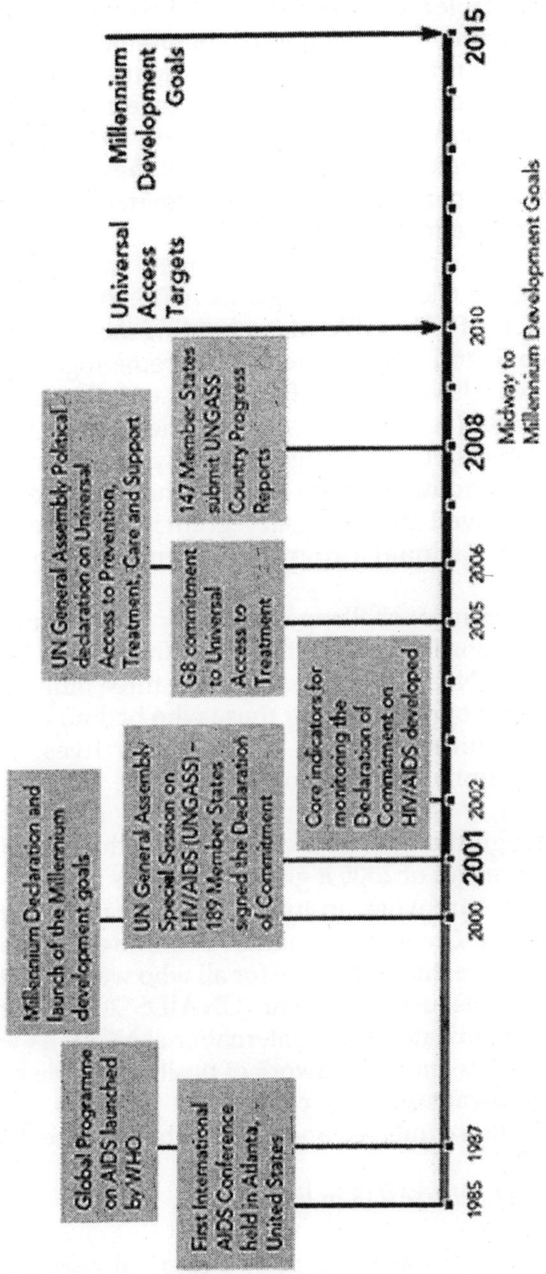

Fig. 5.1: Selected Events in Global Response to the Epidemic

Source: 2008 Report on the Global AIDS Epidemic, *www.unaids.org*, retrieved on 20.4.2009.

that access to affordable medicines for HIV/AIDS was becoming bleak.[1] At this juncture the international community started to lobby to bring down the price of these essential drugs by negotiating and advocating with different governments and NGOs. These endeavours bore fruit when there was a modification in the patent laws, subsequently the price of the essential drugs and particularly the antiretroviral drugs was brought down to an affordable level.

The second most important development has been the establishment of the Global Fund against AIDS, Tuberculosis and Malaria (GFATM). The GFATM is a funding mechanism to fight the epidemic and many nations have come together to fund the GFATM. Although the GFATM was usually short of the required budget (as the national governments have failed to fulfil their pledges) it was a huge leap forward to confront the epidemic. Its funding methods ensured that the countries most-at-need received the necessary grants from them to strengthen their national programmes and control the epidemic.

One of the prominent challenges posed by the epidemic is to treat those millions infected by the virus. In the year 2003, WHO along with UNAIDS set a goal to 'treat three million by 2005.' It was a great opportunity for those who had no chance of getting the required drugs to prolong their lives. This initiative had an immediate positive effect. The number of people receiving antiretroviral increased in a number of countries. Although the desired goal of treating three million was not met by the end of 2005 it gave an impetus to generate political will for future work. In July 2005, the leaders of the G8 countries at the Gleneagles Summit committed to make universal access to treatment by 2010 for all who were infected by HIV/AIDS and needed treatment (UNAIDS 2006). Other developmental organizations and international NGOs as well as the national NGOs and the network of positive people have also played significant roles to control the progress of the disease and help those infected and affected by the disease.

National Response to HIV/AIDS in India

National governments have also been a cardinal part of the

whole in fighting the dreaded disease. They have been quick to react to the dangers posed by the epidemic and put programmes in place to confront it. In India, National AIDS Committee was formed as the report of the first case of HIV was reported. Soon the establishment of NACO followed suit. NACO was given the responsibility to formulate and implement policies and programmes to effectively control and prevent the spread of HIV/AIDS in India. The states were also encouraged to formulate their own strategies to confront the epidemic. Initially, India lacked both knowledge and resources to confront the epidemic. Medium Term Plan was formulated as soon as the first case of HIV/AIDS surfaced. By the year 1992 NACO had formulated the first National AIDS Control Programme (NACP). It had some gaps which needed to be addressed soon in order to make the programme effective in controlling and preventing the spread of HIV/AIDS. In the subsequent NACP II (1999-2006) the gaps which existed in NACP I were identified and attempts were made to rectify them. The lessons learned during NACP I were incorporated in NACP II. With the changing dynamics of the epidemic and with the lessons learnt and achievements made during the earlier two programmes, NACO has now formulated NACP III for the control and prevention of the epidemic and for the treatment, care and support of those infected by the disease. With the growing complexity of the epidemic, there have been changes in the policy framework and approaches of the NACP. Focus has shifted from raising awareness to behavioural change, from a national response to a decentralized response and an increasing engagement of NGOs and networks of PLWHA. Further, the establishment of the States AIDS Control Societies has helped to decentralize the control and prevention programme of NACO thus helping it to reach areas beyond it had earlier envisaged. A great political will was also shown by India to control and prevent HIV/AIDS with the formation of National Council on AIDS chaired by the Prime Minister.

Civil societies have also played a prominent role in preventing the spread of the virus. NGOs and CBOs have been the bridge between the government and the people in the fight against the epidemic. Where the government mechanisms have failed they have been able to take the message of HIV/AIDS to the people. The NGOs and CBOs are more amenable to the public than the government due to the bureaucratic nature, the power and hierarchy involved in governmental mechanism. Instances of NGOs' exemplary contribution to the control and prevention of the epidemic as well as treatment support and care for those infected and affected by the epidemic can be found in plenty in the literature of the disease. Some of the organizations which have been exemplary are YRG Care, Naz Foundation and Lawyer's Collective. YRG Care was the pioneer in providing care and treatment to those infected by HIV/AIDS. Naz Foundation was the first to work among the MSM and the Lawyers Collective was the first to fight legal battles in favour of the PLWHA.

In Darjeeling, lately there has been an escalation in the number of HIV/AIDS cases. As the health sector is not equipped to provide the necessary services, both medical and psycho-social, to those infected by the virus the civil societies have come forward to help the PLWHA. Shanker Foundation, a network of the positive people has come in the forefront to advocate the issues that needs to be dealt for the progress of the PLWHA. This section introduces some of the NGOs and institutions working in the field of HIV/AIDS in the hills of Darjeeling. It also gives us a broad picture of their activities and an account of the funding structure of the NGOs.

Institutional Response of Selected Organisations and Institutions in Darjeeling

In most of the countries, early civil society initiatives are the foundations on which the national responses have been built. It is civil society which remains at the forefront of prevention, care and support programmes, particularly among the most vulnerable and hard to reach populations (UNAIDS 2006). The civil society is uniquely placed to help ensure a long-term perspective to HIV/AIDS. This section deals with the responses HIV/AIDS has received from different institutions in Darjeeling hills.

Medical Institutions

As in other parts of India and West Bengal, the Darjeeling

district hospital is one of the main components of the agency controlling and preventing HIV/AIDS in the hills of Darjeeling. The district hospital is supported by the sub-divisional hospitals at Kurseong and Kalimpong.

The VCCTC which is the primary component of HIV/AIDS control and prevention was started in the district hospital on 1st April, 2002. A spectrum of behaviour change communication initiatives were undertaken to motivate those people who come there and indulge in risk behaviour. Its primary function is to provide pre- and post-test counselling to all the clients who come there. During the pre-test counselling a rapport building exercise is undertaken by the counsellor. After a good rapport is built, the risks are identified. The clients are advised on all the risks and also advised on how to lead a healthy life, if tested positive. The test is not undertaken until and unless the clients are ready psychologically and they duly fill in and sign the consent form. For the clients who test positive, post-test counselling is imparted. The post-test counselling concentrates on behaviour change of the infected individual and also deals with providing psychological support. However, it is more on paper than in practice. They are also advised to go to Shanker Foundation for greater emotional and psychological support.

The VCCTC also started the prevention of parent to child transmission (PPTCT) on 18th March, 2006. Prevention of parent to child transmission of HIV can occur during pregnancy, at the time of delivery or through breastfeeding. However, PPTCT can be done with a combination of short-term drugs treatment, safe delivery practices, counselling and support and safe infant feeding methods. All the pregnant mothers are counselled on HIV/AIDS and are tested for it if they are willing to get themselves tested. After testing if an expectant mother is found positive she is put under the programme. The mother is provided with ART till the time she gives birth and the child is provided with the ART till the age of 18 months to prevent the virus from being transmitted.

The VCCTC at the district hospital also provides facility for post-exposure prophylaxis. Though the district hospital provides the facility for testing, counselling, prevention of parent to child transmission and post-exposure prophylaxis, they do not provide any facility for care and support and counting of CD4 cells and also do not provide any ART to the PLWHA in the hospital. Today to be infected with HIV is no longer synonymous with death because a person with HIV can survive for many years more than previously possible, provided that they receive all necessary treatment and care. Life and death depends to a large extent on one's access to ART which is mediated by the state through hospitals and market institutions. ART is expensive for a poor person who is infected with HIV, as is the case for most PLWHA in Darjeeling. So the State has become the factor which will decide the life or death for the PLWHA. If the state provides free or subsidized ART then these people can prolong their life (Masanjala 2007). But in a situation where the state cannot provide such medicines then many will not be able to afford the high cost of medicine and subsequently succumb to the virus. Unfortunately, the Darjeeling district hospital does not provide ART to the PLWHA.

The hospitals in Kurseong and Kalimpong and also the district hospital have a blood bank and the blood is screened for HIV/AIDS. These hospitals also have STI/STD clinic but the number of people going there are very few as the staff lack sensitivity towards the patients. The hospitals also do not have trained staff who could take care of the PLWHA. As most of the respondents from the study area reported, *"that the hospitals lack the basic facilities and for anything serious one has to go to Siliguri."*

Though the district hospital is doing some work with the ultimate goal of preventing the spread of HIV/AIDS, it has a lot of gaps which need to be plugged. The sexual health awareness among the people is low and not much is being done to improve the knowledge of the community members, women in particular. The STI/RTI is not addressed and many are not utilizing the public sector for its treatment but are instead opting for private treatment. The district health department should in collaboration with the NGOs and CBOs conduct awareness campaigns on sexual health for both men and women addressing the problems of RTI/STI and its linkage with HIV/AIDS. In doing so they should also encourage the people to use condoms and come to the VCCTC.

NGOs they do not have any inclination for the control and prevention of the epidemic. None of the schools in the hills have sex education as a part of their curriculum. One of the principals of a school said, *"We do not have any sex education in the school as most of the students are young and do not understand sex."* In terms of HIV/AIDS, the schools do not have any programmes of their own but some NGOs do go to the schools and give lectures on HIV/AIDS. But this is only done in the few high schools in urban areas and the colleges and other schools are left out.

The majority of the young people in the sample do not have much knowledge about how HIV/AIDS is transmitted or how one can protect against HIV/AIDS. These people become sexually active quite early in life and are likely to use the services of the high risk groups. Under such circumstances it becomes imperative for the authorities to reach out to these young cohorts early in life and teach them to become responsible and to impart correct knowledge of safe sex. The educational institutions have the best reach among such people. Though the School AIDS Education Programme is now being implemented across India by the Department of Education in collaboration with and supported by the SACS (NACO), the schools, both secondary and higher secondary, have not yet implemented this programme in their curriculum in the Darjeeling hills.

The Political Institutions

The political leaders at the district and the community levels have the capacity to mobilize people as they are in constant touch with them. They are at a vantage point for disseminating information on HIV/AIDS as their reach is broader and wider than many NGOs. Due to their importance in the local hierarchy they can lend authority to programmes, influence individuals and groups to change behaviour and generate a positive and supportive environment for the vulnerable population (NACO 2006). Since the political parties control the trade unions they can educate the workforce. As the workforce generally involves the heads of the families they can in turn educate other family members on prevention, care and support.

The political institutions of Darjeeling are not involved in the control and prevention of HIV/AIDS. Due to the non-functioning of the DGHC and the renewed demand for Gorkhaland the political parties have other political agendas and do not involve themselves in the prevention and control of HIV/AIDS. One political leader who the researcher wanted to interview denied giving an interview saying that HIV/AIDS was not his concern and it came under the purview of the health department. Others too did not want to be interviewed on the issue of HIV/AIDS. The political parties are insensitive and unaware of the dangers posed by HIV/AIDS. The political leaders from the grass root up to the higher level are not mobilizing the community for HIV/AIDS awareness programmes. One of the respondents said, *"The politicians can play a big part in checking the spread of HIV/AIDS. If they involve themselves then they can make a huge difference. If they get involved then the Gram Panchayats and other political institutions will also get involved and it becomes easier to reach the grass root."* The only involvement of the political institutions is through the DGHC, which has one of secretaries as the executive member of the DACC. However, this limited involvement of the DGHC is also obstructed to a large extent because of the non-functioning of the DGHC.

The councillors of the municipalities were also found to be ignorant about HIV/AIDS. They do not have any programmes for HIV/AIDS. They are very insensitive to the demands of HIV/AIDS. One of the councillors said, *"HIV/AIDS can be controlled easily. We can organize a mass blood donation camp and identify those who are HIV positive and cull them. This way we can know who are positive and break all ties with them and they will slowly vanish."* Most of the political leaders were also not interested to give interview regarding HIV/AIDS. The Panchayats also do not have any programmes for HIV/AIDS. The non-functioning of DGHC has put an enormous pressure on the NGOs as the funds coming to DACC are delayed thereby delaying further disbursement.

Shanker Foundation: A Network of Positive People

The most prominent institutions working in the field of HIV/

AIDS in the hills of Darjeeling is the Shanker Foundation. Shanker Foundation was formed in 2005 as Shrishti, under the guidance of Kripa AIDS Cell, an arm of Kripa Foundation. It was formally registered under the West Bengal Societies Act only as late as 2006. But now it has evolved on its own and is the only foundation run by PLWHA in Darjeeling. It is a network of positive people and currently has 56 members of which 22 are females and the rest 34 are males. It tries to address the concerns of the positive people with its limited financial as well as human resources. The foundation has been reaching out to PLWHA who have very little means of support. The challenge of constant care and support to the increasing number of people living with the disease is a daunting task for the foundation.

There are many issues that Shanker Foundation is working on, although it is in its infancy. There is a lack of technical help and the positive members themselves have to work in addressing these issues which it considers to be pressing and important. Among other things they face social stigma and discrimination. It is apparent that social stigma and discrimination is a major impediment for them as only 5 of their members have declared their positive status and all the organizational work rests on their shoulders.

Lack of resources and trained personnel within their organization is also a major limitation for them as the number of positive people is increasing and the VCCTC sends all those who are tested positive to the foundation for further counselling, care, treatment and support. However, they are not provided with any financial support by the VCCTC. This in addition with the insufficient medical support also puts a lot of pressure on the foundation to meet with the aspirations and hope of those who are sent there by the VCCTC. The plight of the PLWHA is further accentuated as the doctors, nurses and other health staff do not show any sensitivity towards the conditions of the PLWHA.

Under such adverse conditions Shanker Foundation has till date carried out a number of activities which have helped at least a handful of people if not all. The most important activity undertaken by the Shanker Foundation has been to encourage five of its members to disclose their positive status to the public and give a face to the HIV/AIDS problems in the hills. Simultaneously, it has brought to the notice of the public that everybody is in the danger of being infected by HIV and that there are numerous problems faced by the PLWHA. Prior to this there was no one whom the public knew to be HIV positive. It was generally held that HIV/AIDS was a 'western disease' and that they would not be affected or infected by it.

As there is no formal care and support system in the hills of Darjeeling for the PLWHA the members of the Foundation are working overtime to provide care and support to all those who are positive and come there willingly. On a day to day basis Shanker Foundation provides care and support to positive people within the network through counselling, family visits (for only the members who have disclosed their status to the family) and trainings. The counselling and training is focused on enhancing life skills of positive people and their families.

Along with providing counselling and training to those who are positive it is also trying to strengthen and expand its member base. As many of the individuals who test positive do not come to the Foundation (out of the 141 tested positive only 56 are its members) they are persuading those positive people to come to the Foundation and be a part of it. In this endeavour they are attempting to expand their network to Kurseong, Kalimpong and Mirik.

Although the foundation lacks in financial resources, it provides nutritional support to its members who are economically weak. In this activity another organization, Friends supports them. Though they are providing nutritional support to many of their members they require more financial support from the DACC as they can afford only rupees twenty five per member per month. They are aware that this amount can give them nothing which is nutritious for even a day.

To monitor the care and support given by the Foundation a meeting is held every Saturday. The members are encouraged to talk and give inputs so that the Foundation can improve on their work. For sensitizing the families of the PLWHA every month a meeting is held with the families (who know about their family member's health) who are affected by HIV/AIDS and are sensitized to care and support the PLWHA. In this endeavour, the volunteers from Friends play an important role as they make it evident with their participation that non-positive people need to take active part in the well-being of the positive people.

Though the Shanker Foundation is doing so much for the welfare of the PLWHA, they lack in networking as the members do not have any training in running an organisation. Most of the PLWHA are not well educated and this acts as an impediment in their effort to network. The members of the Foundation were also not adept at advocacy as they are not aware of many related issues. Only recently they have started joining hands with other organizations of PLWHA or those working for the welfare of the PLWHA. Due to their lack of awareness of the legislative developments they were found wanting with regards to the laws protecting the rights of the PLWHA.

FRIENDS—Sister Concern of Shanker Foundation

This organization is the backbone to Shanker Foundation. It was started in 2002 when a number of like minded people came together to confront the menace of HIV/AIDS. It is a group of volunteers who work within the Shanker Foundation. They are the helping hand required by Shanker Foundation. The co-coordinator of the organization narrates the story of how Friends came into existence.

It started as 'Shristi' in 2002 under the guidance of Kripa AIDS Cell. Most of the members of Shanker Foundation were IDUs. One day, unfortunately one of the members of the Shanker Foundation died and a memorial service was held when the coordinator prayed. She said she thought "I have the heart so why don't I do something for them." She had been hearing a lot about HIV/AIDS and the problems faced by the PLWHA. She had seen people dying of HIV/AIDS and how they were ill treated. They were kept on the floor and left to die. Then people did not know much about HIV/AIDS.

They helped the PLWHA to find space for the present day office of Shanker Foundation. Then awareness campaigns were started by printing brochures and pamphlets. After Shanker Foundation was established with its office, they opened a saving account in the UTI bank in the name of Shanker Foundation.

Most of the volunteers started to contribute and though efforts were made to collect funds from other sources as well, it was not very successful. Eventually funds started coming from people who were conscious of HIV/AIDS and though it helped to a large extent it was insufficient.

'Friends' provide emotional, psychological and nutritional support to the members of the Foundation. They are not just confined to supporting the PLWHA but also work with the families of those infected. It is very important for them to work with the families as the DACC does not provide any support to the families of the PLWHA. Apart from this they also go to visit the hospitals with the PLWHA when they need any medical intervention. They try to make sure that none of the PLWHA carry any opportunistic infections. If any of the PLWHA has OI they take them to the appropriate hospital. They have collaborated with Planter's Hospital in Darjeeling. To get the CD4 cell counted they take the PLWHA to NBMCH whenever necessary as well as those who need to collect the ARVs.

'Friends', as an organization also makes sure that the funds are disbursed to Shanker Foundation on time. Earlier there were funds coming but not a single penny was granted to Shanker Foundation. 'Friends' have constantly fought for the grants and since 2006 funds are coming to the Foundation through the DACC. As there is a dual government of the DGHC and West Bengal there is a lot of problem regarding the smooth flow of the grants to the Shanker Foundation. Shanker Foundation has received grants 3-4 times but Friends had to struggle for these grants. They are at times harassed and have to go through a lot of bureaucratic hassle in getting the funds. Recently an advocate has joined 'Friends' and she has committed to help them with the legal provisions. She is the human rights advisor and with her help and advice 'Friends' is fighting those who discriminate against the PLWHA.

As most of the PLWHA are from the economically weaker section of the society they are trying to start an income generation scheme. They are at the moment trying to start with knitting, as the number of female PLWHA is also large. They are also negotiating with the business community to sell their products. Once this starts the economic problem can be solved to a large extent.

Sewa Karya—a Darjeeling Based NGO

'Sewa Karya' is a non-profit non-governmental organization established in 1999. It is a subsidiary of the West Bengal Voluntary Health Association and its projects are funded by the state. It also receives fund from some corporate sectors as well as from the DACC.

'Sewa Karya' has projects on STI/STD and HIV/AIDS. It started the projects in 2000 in Ging Tea Estate with HIV/AIDS programme for the workers of tea industry. Initially, the project received mixed reaction from the local populace. The first year of the programme was a struggle as there was no support from the people but in the second year there was greater cooperation.

Working in the tea garden has given them a lot of experience, particularly in the area of STI and STD. While working among the tea garden workers they received a lot of cases of STI and STD among both the men and women but the maximum cases were detected among the women as the men were reluctant to visit the STI/STD clinic they had started. Under their guidance and counselling all those who were infected with STI and STD were advised for HIV testing. To their dismay many were found to be HIV positive. They had thought of the test as a precautionary method but the number of those who were found to be positive baffled them.

After 3 years the sponsors stopped funding the programme but 'Sewa Karya' carried on with the programme till 2005. They had to stop the programme as their parent body also stopped funding the programme. However, they had sent a proposal for a programme on tea garden workers and their spouses. At the moment they engage themselves with the workers of the tea estate by organizing workshops on health and hygiene and family planning.

At present they are conducting a home based care for the PLWHA which is sponsored by their parent body WBVHA. This programme is the first of its kind in the hills of Darjeeling. In this endeavour they are aided by a counsellor and a field worker. In this programme the 'Sewa Karya' provides 4 services to benefit the PLWHA.

- Psychological Service (counselling) to the PLWHA and their family members.
- Emergency Medical Support
- Nutritional Support and
- Social Support

Psychological Services: Most of the PLWHA are not highly educated and there is hardly any post-counselling available, so it becomes imperative for the non-governmental organizations to provide some post-counselling. There have been instances where the PLWHA have acted irresponsibly and therefore there is a need for counselling the PLWHA. As the family members of the PLWHA play a salient role in the latter's well-being it is necessary for them to be well informed. Apart from this, the family members need counselling as they may also discriminate against the PLWHA.

Emergency Medical Support: Many of the PLWHA in the hills of Darjeeling come from economically weaker category and therefore do not have much resource to spend on OIs. Some may even postpone the required treatment. This support is to ensure that the OIs are not neglected by the PLWHA. 'Sewa Karya' makes sure that the medical expenditure is reimbursed to the PLWHA who have sought treatment for the OIs or had the OIs treated. The 'Sewa Karya' however, follows a strict regulation for the reimbursement of the medical bills. The PLWHA have to show the staff of the 'Sewa Karya' the prescription of the doctor and the amount spent on the prescribed medicine is reimbursed after verification of the receipt. Apart from providing financial support for medicines 'Sewa Karya' also provides physical care to those PLWHA who have been hospitalized. Volunteers of the organization provide care to the sick PLWHA.

Nutritional Support: Nutritional support is provided to only those PLWHA who have been adopted by the organization. They were providing this facility to very few PLWHA at the time of field visit. Due to the financial constraints they had adopted only a few PLWHA but they intend to adopt more PLWHA in the future when they get more funds.

Social Support: This support is provided by 'Sewa Karya' to fight discrimination against the PLWHA. Due to the lack of adequate knowledge of HIV/AIDS people still discriminate the PLWHA. 'Sewa Karya' is trying to raise awareness among the public to curb the discrimination. Whenever there is a case of discrimination the volunteers from 'Sewa Karya' go to the spot and conduct awareness programmes to ensure that such acts of discrimination does not occur in the future. They also make an effort to engage the local community in this endeavour.

MANAS (MSM Advocacy Network for Social Action) Bangla, Darjeeling

MANAS Bangla Darjeeling is a part of the national NGO MANAS Bangla. It primarily works on the issues relating to MSM. It started functioning in the hills of Darjeeling when HIV/AIDS cases started to rise in the hills. It did not get the support it required initially. They work with a marginalized group which is often ridiculed by others. They were even accused of encouraging unwanted behaviour among the youth. It started to function during adverse conditions and today has a drop-in centre at Kurseong and Darjeeling. The organization says that there are more than 500 MSM in the hills and they have started work to promote safe sexual behaviour among this group of marginalized people and reduce the transmission of HIV/AIDS among this group.

The objective of the organization has been to promote sexual health and safe sexual practices among the MSM in the hills of Darjeeling and also reduce the incidence of HIV among the group. They are progressing towards their goal with the targeted intervention project currently being carried out in Darjeeling and Kurseong. Their focus has been to bring about behavioural changes among the MSM in their sexual practices. They encourage the MSM to bring the change through behaviour change communication, treatment support for any infection that MSM get from their sexual practices. They encourage the MSM to use condoms and lubricants. The organization is also working to bring about a change in the attitude of the people regarding the MSM and built an environment where the MSM are not castigated because of their sexual orientation.

They are conducting the Programme Integrated Darjeeling Hills Male to Male Sexual Health Promotion and HIV Control are based on the four principles:

- Awareness and capacity building through peer education, condom and lubricant promotion.
- STD/HIV/AIDS counselling, testing, treatment and related counselling and referrals.
- Creation of enabling environment.
- Behaviour change communication development and dissemination and community mobilization and networking among them and capacity building.

The MSM population is invisible in the hills as it is in many regions. The organization faced a difficult proposition to identify them and bring them into their folds. In order to reach as many MSM as possible they recruited other MSM as peer educators and outreach workers. They were trained and sent to the field to identify and recruit MSM in their programme. After the initial difficulties today MANAS Bangla is working with more than 100 MSM.

These outreach workers identify and bring the MSM to the office where the peer educator imparts them with the knowledge and advantages of safe sex, STD/HIV/AIDS. The MSM are encouraged to ask questions and inquire about various issues concerning themselves. The MSM who come to the centre are encouraged to use condoms and lubricants. To make them use these aids was a major hindrance as they held contrary beliefs to the use of such devices. As the convener of a drop-in centre said, *"They did not believe that they could get infected with HIV/AIDS when we started counselling the first few MSM who came here. Further those who agreed to try condoms and lubricants complained saying that using condom obstructed their sexual act and tore the skin. However, they were in favour of the lubricants. Although after a lot of convincing they have started to use condoms. Now they complain that the condoms reduce the pleasure of sex."*

The MSM in the hills were oblivious to the risk of HIV/AIDS and STD due to their unsafe sexual practices thereby rendering counselling very important. Everyday those MSM who come to the centre are counselled about STD/HIV/AIDS. The counselling is rigorous and sustained till the individual is fully aware of STD/HIV/AIDS and the benefits of condom use and safe sex practices. Group discussions are also held among them so that they learn and engage themselves in the dissemination of knowledge about STD and HIV/AIDS. Positive people from Shanker Foundation are also invited to address them so that they can learn more about their experiences and the infection.

Treatment is also imparted to those MSM who have any STD. They are counselled and treatment is provided locally by a doctor employed by the organization. However, this facility is available only when the doctor comes to the centre after the completion of his/her duty. Medication required for the treatment of the STD is also available at the office of the organization. In case the STD/STI is acute, referral arrangements are made by MANAS Bangla and then the individual is encouraged to get tested for HIV, the arrangements for which are also made by the organization. In the advent of such a situation pre- and post-counselling is also provided by the organization.

Community mobilization is done with the help of the peer educators. They in partnership with MANAS Bangla work among the MSM of Darjeeling. The MSM are mobilized and an enabling environment is created where they can articulate their views and ideas pertaining to their experiences. The member of the community are advised and encouraged to meet and discuss and disseminate the knowledge of safe sex, STD/HIV/AIDS. Through many training programmes the capacity and skills of the MSM are developed.

Today MANAS Bangla has two drop-in centres one each at Darjeeling and Kurseong. The drop-in centres are open everyday except Sunday. The centres provide the facility of face to face counselling with the counsellor. They also conduct Group discussion, condom demonstration and video shows.

Both the drop-in centres have STI clinic to diagnose and treat STIs and STDs by a doctor and the counsellor provides pre- and post-test counselling. The clinic facilitates the process of HIV testing for patients by referring them to the VCCTC.

Workshops and seminars are also organized for advocacy and sensitization of the general population, students, other NGOs and the police on the issues of MSM.

The Indian Red Cross Society, Kurseong

At the district level there is a 13 member Managing Committee with the District Magistrate as the Chairman and the Chief Medical Officer as the Vice-Chairman of the IRCS. The Sub-Divisional Officer is the Ex-Officio Chairman of the society.

As the prevalence among the IDUs is one of the highest in the state of West Bengal, IRCS has started a targeted intervention programme for the prevention of HIV/AIDS among the IDUs and the shadow users.[2] The programme is aided by trained peer counsellors and outreach workers who are also former IDUs and this makes the implementation of the programme easier as these peer educators and outreach workers can relate to the IDUs more convincingly and emphatically. The programme is conducted through the Harm Reduction Network called 'Kalyan.' Under this network drop-in centres at Kurseong, Darjeeling and Kalimpong were started where harm reduction intervention by providing Needle Syringe Exchange Programme (NSEP) and Drug Substitution Therapy (DST) were carried out. At present there are five drop-in centres, two more have been recently started in Mirik and Ghoom. The programme was initially funded by the DFID through an organization called 'Sharan' based in New Delhi. The programme is today funded by the State AIDS Control and Prevention Society through the DACC. Apart from providing NSEP and DST using Buprenorphine at these drop-in centres, medical care by a doctor, counselling by a trained counsellor, abscess management by a trained nurse, free referrals for HIV testing and further treatment is extended. Till the time of data collection the network was providing services to more than 1200 drug dependent in hills of Darjeeling.

This harm reduction programme is amenable to the IDUs and other drug dependents as services are provided free of cost and by trained personnel, it does not require hospitalization and one can carry on with their daily chores while on treatment and it also helps to prevent HIV/AIDS. As the clients have to attend the clinic daily they are in constant touch with the members of the clinic who boost their morale and address their needs. While on field visits the peer educators also counsel the family members along with the clients thereby involving the family members in the well being of their clients. This also gives the client a sense of being loved and feeling cared for.

The process of harm reduction in the drop-in centres entails a number of steps before one is provided with the services. It is a step by step process. At first the client has to go through a one-to-one session with the counsellor. During this process the counsellor gets to know about the history of the client, his personality, family background, medical history as well as the history of his/her drug addiction. In the process the client is made aware of the dangers of injecting drugs and the different options that are available to him/her that could potentially free him/her from drug addiction and also prevent from being infected by HIV/AIDS. At this stage the counsellor introduces the client to NSEP and DST.

The client is given the choice of whether or not he/she wants to quit the habit of drugs. After they give their consent the client is examined by a doctor. The doctor while medically examining the client thoroughly assesses his/her degree of drug dependence. According to the degree of the client's drug dependence, the doctor decides whether the client needs medication or can be weaned out only with counselling. Simultaneously, the client is also educated in safe sex practices and condoms are provided free to the clients as per the individual's need and requirement. Apart from this the spouse, if any and the family is also counselled.

In cases where the client refuses to stop the habit of injecting drugs, they are informed of all the dangers of injecting drugs such as abscess formation, collapse of veins, infection of the heart and kidneys, transmission of HIV/AIDS. The clients are then counselled to adopt safer infection practices like not sharing needles and syringes, use of new syringe needles for each injection, use of sterilized syringe needles in case one is not available and injecting safely and at relatively safer places to prevent complications such as police harassment. Under the NSEP such clients are provided new needles and syringes free against deposit of the used ones. The outreach workers and peer educators closely monitor the NSEP. As the client starts engaging in safer injecting practices he is counselled and assisted to decrease the dose and gradually encouraged to shift to Buprenorphine before making him/her retire from drug dependency.

Again when an IDU after counselling wants to switch to oral Buprenorphine, then the client is thoroughly examined by a doctor to assess whether or not the client is an IDU. After having ascertained the status of the client the doctor assesses the degree of drug dependency. After the intensity of drug addiction is ascertained the client is put under a supervised oral Buprenorphine regime. The IDU starts with 2 mg Buprenorphine and is subsequently reduced with the advice of the doctor. The minimum dose of Buprenorphine is 0.2 mg which is administered when it is ascertained that the client is in a position to quit drugs. After this dose administration of Buprenorphine is totally stopped so that the client becomes independent of drug injecting habit.

Apart from these interventions, the IRCS also provides referral services to the drop-in centres. The drop-in centres also provide financial support for the treatment of the oral drug users in rehabilitation and detoxification centres. These initiatives are taken by the IRCS anticipating that the oral drug users can shift to injecting drug use within a short span of time. Throughout the period of referral to the admission to the detoxification centre and the release from the detoxification centre the staff from the drop-in centres constantly interact with the clients and their family members and provide support to enable the individual to lead a drug free life.

The project 'Kalyan' has taken up the challenge to prevent HIV transmission among the IDUs and from them to the community. They have taken this initiative by trying to enable the IDUs to lead a drug free life and thereby integrating them in the society, as meaningful citizens.

Himalayan Anti AIDS and Narcotic Drugs Society (HANDS), Kalimpong

HANDS, is an organization which is trying to spread awareness on HIV/AIDS and at the same time tackle the exponential rise of drug abuse in Kalimpong sub-division. It was started in June 2006 by a group of prominent citizens of Kalimpong. The main objectives of HANDS are:

- To organize training facilities, seminars and workshops in order to disseminate information on AIDS and drug abuse as a part of adult education programmes and as a part of school AIDS and drug abuse education programme.
- To provide counselling to drug/alcohol addicts and their families in order to help them deal with their addiction.
- To conduct therapeutic input sessions among the addicts.
- To conduct outreach programmes, i.e. to reach addicts at their homes and streets in order to bring them to the day care centre.
- In the long-term, to set up a Rehabilitation Centre at Kalimpong where addicts from the sub-division may obtain treatment at the most affordable rates.

In order to fulfil their objectives, the HANDS team has conducted awareness lectures in a number of schools at Kalimpong. This is a sustained and constant endeavour of HANDS as they realize the importance of educating the students who are young and vulnerable. Their focus has not been limited to students alone. They also conduct outreach programmes among the drug and alcohol dependent persons. Due to this effort almost 100 drug abusers have been motivated till the day of interview to come to the day care centre to receive counselling and therapeutic inputs. These counselling and therapeutic inputs are imparted session-wise, judging the requirement of those coming there.

Adult education on AIDS and drug abuse has been the cornerstone of their success and it is being pursued vigorously. As there are few organizations imparting adult education this endeavour has become a very salient component of their programmes. Though not much interest has been shown by the public and at times they had to face adversity they are still pursuing with their goals. Sessions on adult education is carried out in the Town Hall and everybody who comes there is provided with information, education and communication materials.

They also have a referral service whereby chronic drug dependent persons are referred to some rehabilitation centres. The drug dependent persons are also counselled to undergo HIV testing. If the person gives his or her consent to undergo HIV testing then the individual is referred to the VCCTC.

Family's Response to HIV/AIDS in Darjeeling

The number of care givers in the sample is very less (5) and comprises only 2.51 per cent. There were 4 females and one male. The females were between 23 and 45 years and the only male care giver was 38 years old. Among the 4 female care givers one was a wife of an infected person, two were mothers and one was a niece of an infected person. 4 of the care givers heard about HIV/AIDS only after their wards were diagnosed to be HIV positive. The main concern of the care givers was to prolong the life of the infected person. Their endeavour was however challenged by the stigmatization and discriminating nature of the infection. They were in complete shock on hearing that their wards were HIV positive.

The care givers who were present at the time of the disclosure of the test result have been supportive of the PLWHA and have not disclosed their sero status. The care givers were scared of losing their family members. The care givers were also equally concerned about keeping the status of their wards a secret as they were intimidated by the discrimination and subsequent isolation of their wards. A care giving woman said, *"I have not disclosed the sero status of my son as he can be discriminated and along with him also the family can be discriminated. We have to protect him otherwise he will be left with nobody for support."* The care givers were also motivated to care and support their infected family member as they have come to know that only proper care and emotional support can prolong their life. The wife of a PLWHA said, *"The doctor told me that there is no cure for this disease, but if we keep him happy and not let him know that he will ultimately die, then he can live longer. So I have taken upon myself not to let him die an unhappy death and provide him with all the care and support he needs."*

Most of the PLWHA were asymptomatic at the time of interview but with the onset of full blown AIDS the care givers have to provide care during the time when they fall ill and provide good nutritious food, monitor their health, diet and lifestyles and importantly provide them the emotional support they need and accompany them to the hospital whenever required. One of the care givers said, *"I do not have to do much as my daughter does not have any illness now. But the important thing for me now is to check that she eats her food regularly and is not disturbed by fears of death as there is no medicine. I have to make sure that she is not suffering from any illness and her health is good."* Another woman said, *"The most important thing for me now is to make sure that my son does not indulge in drug abuse and eats properly. I have to make sure that he is enjoying his life in his own way and is not preoccupied with unnecessary thoughts. It must be difficult for him but I try to make his life as easy as possible and provide him all the support he needs. I try to make him understand that he is loved by the family and we do not have anything against him."* She further adds, *"The fact that there is no medicine to cure this disease and he will die made me forget all the troubles he had put us into, and care for him. This way I help him to repose faith in us as we were very upset about his behaviour earlier and blamed his behaviour for acquiring HIV. If I can care for him now then may be God will forgive me for cursing him all those days when he used to trouble us due to his drug addiction."* Another care giver said, *"I had to care for my friend as there is only his old mother who cannot do anything. It was my moral duty to care for him as we have done all the things together whether, acceptable or not. It was just my good luck that I am not infected by HIV. The fact is there is not much to do as well. I go spend some time with him and see that he is eating properly and keeping good health. Earlier I used to accompany him to the hospital but now this is also taken care by Shanker Foundation. I try to see that he is not depressed and emotionally disturbed."*

The experiences of the affected people revolved around the desire to prolong the life of their kins and the fear of losing them. Most of the respondents thought that it was their duty to care for the infected person though they were also concerned about the economic aspect of care giving when the asymptomatic condition would turn into full blown AIDS. Most of the respondents were aware of the economic resources that were available to them and that they would not be able to deal with the disease with the existing resources. One of the respondents said, *"My daughter is HIV positive but she is not ill, so there is not much expenditure on medicines at the moment. But once her condition deteriorates it will be very difficult to take care of her as we do not have much money. We have to look after others as well and cannot spend all the income on her medicines. This thought troubles me a lot, all the time, as I know a time will come when she will need a lot of care and medicines. Neither can we overlook her medicinal needs nor can we overlook the expenditure on other things."* Most of the care givers, however, were determined to give the utmost care and support to the PLWHA even during the times of adversity. Many of the care givers were of the opinion that they would overcome the economic shortcoming with their emotional support.

Discrimination and stigma is prevalent in the society against the PLWHA but the people caring for them are selfless individuals working overtime to prolong the life of their beloved family members and friends. There are many concerns for the care givers but they are determined to provide care as much as they can and provide all the emotional support so that the PLWHA under their supervision do not undergo unnecessary emotional distress.

The Community's Response

The population of Darjeeling hills is composed of people belonging to diverse ethnic communities. The majority of the people primarily belong to the ethnic group Nepali. This ethnic group is divided into the *'Tagedharies'*[3] and the *'Matwalis'*.[4] Though in the hills of Darjeeling caste system or discrimination on the basis of caste is not covert but in matters of marriage it does exists. Due to this various caste based 'samaj'[5] has come into existence, which look after the well-being of its members. They have become an important agent in controlling its members and carrying out some developmental works for the people. They maintain records of their members and the network among the *samaj* of different places is well established. These *samajs* are directly or indirectly involved in one's life from the time of the individual's birth. However, having so much say in the life of the people belonging to the caste, they probably, due to lack of awareness have failed to understand the contribution they can make in the control and prevention of HIV/AIDS. Many sophisticated models of HIV/AIDS prevention and control have recognized that people who know each other can have a great impact on each other's behaviour. Such social influence can amount to a veto power on high risk behaviour in circumstances where people might otherwise engage in risk behaviour (Friedman *et al.* 2005). This is the principle on which the *samaj* function. They have the veto power over its members in a large number of issues and can therefore extend their powers and bring about behavioural changes in their members. They can directly intervene at the community level and emphasize on the direct modification of the individual behaviour. *Samaj* because of its emphasis on 'manipulating the social reinforcers and environmental constraints associated with desired behaviours' (Rhodes and Mallote 1996) can modify the individual risk behaviours.

The *samaj* has social control over its members and can be very effective in spreading information in the forms of leaflets and discussions, enabling individuals to identify their risk behaviours and bringing about changes in the behavioural environment by addressing the risk behaviours of the members. They can most importantly bring about community development by enhancing health by bringing about community change through collective action (Gadd and Goss 2005). The *samajs* can achieve this community development by participation of its members and by sharing experiences. In order to achieve this they can make presentations on factual information about HIV/AIDS, its modes of transmission and control and prevention. They can also discuss feelings about sex and skills for negotiating safe sex and suggest use of condoms among its members. They can achieve total participation of its members by having separate sessions for the male and female members, if they perceive that males and females may not be able to discuss sexual matters together under the same roof.

There is so much these *samajs* can do in terms of HIV/AIDS control and prevention but nobody has realized their potential. None of the *samajs* were involved in any form in the control and prevention of the epidemic in the hills of Darjeeling. The NGOs and especially the DACC must pay utmost attention and involve them as they can reach every individual belonging to a particular caste.

Religious Institutions

Religious institutions worldwide have played important roles in the control and prevention of HIV/AIDS among its followers. As religious beliefs and practices are important in influencing its followers they can take active role in the control and prevention of HIV/AIDS. Major religions of India like Hinduism, Christianity, Buddhism and Islam are followed by the people of Darjeeling. So these religions can play their part in controlling the spread of HIV/AIDS in Darjeeling. Although they can play a vital role, it is seen that only the Christian community is actively participating in the control and prevention of this epidemic. The Christians, participate not directly but through several NGOs of Darjeeling. Some of the prominent NGOs are the Anugalaya Diocese Centre and Kripa Foundation. They have recently been able to open a new care and support centre at Darjeeling, with 10 beds with the financial support from Global Fund, a Geneva based institution. It will have a doctor and two nurses round the clock. This is an effort that has to be appreciated, as the PLWHA of Darjeeling hill were devoid of such facility and had to depend on the facilities provided by the NBMCH, where they had to face a lot of discrimination. Apart from this, their major contribution has been the home visits they conduct to provide the much needed psychological help. However, they undertake this programme only if the concerned person is willing. They also give information on HIV/AIDS during their services and advise people on leading a healthy life.

Media Response

The mass media are certainly the most widespread means to disperse information to the public. It is a powerful tool and can play an important part in disseminating information on HIV/AIDS by generating awareness. However, they are not only a means of information dispersal. Media is also able to shape attitudes and draw attention to certain issues. Thus, they are not only a major factor in determining what the public knows about important issues, but also what the public thinks about them (Cunningham 2005). It can also influence the opinions on HIV/AIDS and give feedback to the agencies which are responsible for formulating policies with regards to HIV/AIDS (NACO 2006). But the media coverage of HIV/AIDS in Darjeeling is negligible. News pertaining to HIV/AIDS in Darjeeling is covered only by the local newspapers and this cannot generate much support for the PLWHA as well as for the organizations working on the issues of HIV/AIDS in Darjeeling at the national level. Local coverage cannot generate much public opinion to force changes in the policies and create policies which are beneficial to the local PLWHA. The local television channels, which has a wide viewership among the locals is not utilized properly. They do not air any programmes on HIV/AIDS. The concerned authorities should tap the potential of these channels in spreading the information and educating the people on HIV/AIDS. The All India Radio which has its station in Kurseong can also be used to spread information. Though the local newspapers, like the *Himalaya Darpan* and *Sunchari* have started reporting on HIV/AIDS on a regular basis but their reporting is just based on the programmes undertaken by some NGOs and is always confined to the statistics. They have failed to understand their efficacy in making the people understand the ways in which it can be transmitted. During the period of fieldwork none of the dailies reported on the economic and political aspects of the epidemic, on care and support needed by the PLWHA and how stigma and discrimination could make the lives of those infected and affected difficult. The pictures accompanying the articles, though there were very few, always seemed to attribute death and suffering to the PLWHA. There were no articles urging the politicians and the government to look into the needs of the PLWHA. The demand for an ART centre in the hills was never covered by the local media. The coverage of the issue in the local media was mostly negative in the sense that the development of medicines, the ART which has been effective in prolonging the lives of those infected by the virus and its availability and the government's endeavour to make it accessible to all, was seldom reported. The press of the hills of Darjeeling needs to be vigilant enough to understand their responsibility and also report that the development in the scientific world has given hope to the PLWHA for a better life and not equate HIV/AIDS with death and suffering as this will put across a negative message in a place and situation where the PLWHA and the vulnerable sub-groups are stigmatized and discriminated.

The Overview of the Response to HIV/AIDS in Darjeeling Hills

It is quite obvious that HIV/AIDS prevention is not a domain of one particular organization, it has to be conducted by more than one institution. Reaching larger numbers of people from all sections of the society, and carrying out effective policy work will depend on the organization's ability to network with one another. Increased collaboration could also facilitate the development of a common language to describe approaches so that practitioners can better understand one another's work. Although some networking does occur through the DACC, the experience in conducting this study has shown that the networking among the different organizations could be significantly improved. Through discussions during the course of the study, it was established that the organizations involved in HIV/AIDS were not aware of others working in the same area. In spite of this, there are glimpses of efforts being made to improve the networking among the different organisations.

Being the funding agency as well as the bridge between the government and the local institutions, confronting the epidemic, DACC is under tremendous pressure to perform. However, the government has failed to understand this and is reflected by the fact that the DACC is understaffed and for most of the executive members the work and responsibility of DACC is additional to their primary profession. As a consequence, the executive members have little time to devote to the functioning of DACC. Because of the lack of staff, the DACC has not been able to generate commitment and sense of urgency among the people and still there is a high degree of denial regarding HIV/AIDS among the community members. The disbursement of funds to other NGOs, working in the hills, has been slow and this has become a major obstacle in responding effectively to the epidemic. The inability of the DACC to release funds on regular basis has generated immense pressure on the NGOs' effective functioning. One official from Shanker Foundation said, *"I have been coming here for the past 5 days but they do not have the cheque ready. I cannot waste my time coming here everyday as I have many other organizational works to do as well."*

There is very little involvement of the other sectors in the prevention, control, care and treatment of HIV/AIDS in the hills of Darjeeling. The tea gardens and the railways which are the major employers here are not involved in the control and prevention of HIV/AIDS. Their effective and sincere involvement in the prevention and control programme can reach a large number of people. In such a situation, the DACC must encourage these two big sectors to get involved. HIV/AIDS largely remains a health programme devoid of any attempt to bring about changes in the social, cultural, political and economic changes, though there are large volumes of literature linking HIV/AIDS to the social, cultural, political and economic conditions of an individual.

In Darjeeling hills there is only targeted intervention among the high risk groups and the community at large which is being infected and affected by the epidemic is being forgotten. Even now it is a taboo to talk about sex and HIV/AIDS in the family. In such a scenario, it becomes necessary for the institutions working in the sphere of HIV/AIDS to also include the community members in all the stages of planning and implementation of the programme so that the entire population is concerned about the adversity which can be brought by the epidemic.

There are many NGOs working in the field of HIV/AIDS in Darjeeling but there is not much networking among them, as a result they are not aware of the programmes of other NGOs and there is a serious gap in communication among them. Though all the NGOs are linked with the DACC and Shanker Foundation, this link is very weak and merely fulfils their professional needs rather than to create stronger collaboration.

The NGOs are linked with DACC for the funds and with the Shanker Foundation to fulfil the principle of GIPA. Communication is a major training challenge to all the NGOs in the hills of Darjeeling. The communication among the NGOs at best can be said to be casual. Because of this there is not much sharing of information and data which hampers the overall future plans and programmes seriously.

All the programmes in the hills of Darjeeling are being funded by DACC. The proposals from the NGOs are scrutinized by the executive members of the DACC, who decide whether or not to fund a programme. Under such circumstances the institutions are carrying out only those programmes which have been conducted elsewhere. They do not undertake custom made programmes to suit local needs as they fear that their proposals may be rejected. The programmes are largely high risk group centric and do not concentrate on the general public. However, working with the high risk groups is a difficult task for the NGOs as many of them are hidden and invisible. The FSW and the MSM or the bisexuals in the hills of Darjeeling cannot be identified and so working with them becomes a challenge for the NGOs. It is more of a challenging proposition for all the institutions working on issues related to HIV/AIDS as there is the absence of an enabling environment for these high risk groups to come forward and avail the services provided by the various institutions. Because of their focus on high risk groups, the NGOs are concentrating only on control and prevention of the epidemic.

In Darjeeling hills all the NGOs are concentrating only on the prevention and control aspect of the epidemic. The rural areas are left out of these prevention and control programmes to a large extent. They do not focus on care and treatment and support facilities and even the VCCTC refers the positive people to Shanker Foundation for care and support. As the intervention from the NGOs is at the level of high risk groups, the NGOs have not focused on the general public and the families of those infected by the virus. The families of the infected persons are not receiving any support from the NGOs and are going through emotional trauma. There is a greater need for intervention from the NGOs at the familial level. As many of the PLWHA have not yet disclosed their status to their families it also becomes difficult for the NGOs to approach them.

Although the number of NGOs in Darjeeling is increasing, their reach is limited only to a small segment of the society. Apart from the IRCS and the drop-in centres of MANAS Bangla and YMDS there are no independent NGOs working in Kurseong town. At the same time, it can be said that a large segment of the society are unaware of the available assistance as most of the intervention programmes have not focused on them.

Notes and References

1. (*www.accessmed-msf.org* 2005).
2. People who predominantly use pills but whenever they have the opportunity to inject drugs they do so.
3. *Tagedharies* are people who traditionally and culturally prohibit alcohol consumption and belong to the higher castes.
4. *Matwalis* are people who are traditionally and culturally alcohol consuming and belong to the middle and lower rung of the caste hierarchy.
5. These *samajs* work for the upliftment of the concerned caste and people belonging to the caste are compulsorily members of the *samaj*.

Chapter VI

Advent and Spread of HIV/AIDS in Darjeeling: Discussion, Findings and Strategies

The first case of HIV/AIDS in Darjeeling was detected after the epidemic had killed millions, destroyed families, ruptured the social fabric of the society and shattered developmental gains made over many years in many parts of the globe. Since then within 5 years the total number of cases detected was 141. It has become a smooth ride for the virus to spread among the people with very little and ineffective effort to control and prevent it from spreading further. The considerable under-reporting of the virus and the denial among the people has further aggravated the problem. The epidemic is not just confined to the individual it infects but its impact can be felt at diverse levels. Starting from the individual it infects, its impact can be felt at the societal levels forcing change on the established norms and values of the society, denting the development gains made over the years. The impact on the government can be tremendous as it has to subsidize the medicine and other required medical facilities (Gupta *et al.* 2003).

The prevalence of HIV/AIDS is low in the Darjeeling hills. However, this is not an assurance that the situation will be sustained and there will be no further increase in the number of HIV/AIDS cases. The indicators are very fertile for the spread of HIV/AIDS. The virus is found among the IDUs, housewives and children. There is unfortunately a likelihood that it can spread further, before the policy-makers can realize, due to the inadequate infrastructure, the social environment of stigma and discrimination, drug and substance abuse, low rate of condom use and incidences of unsafe sexual practices among the people.

Discussion

The PLWHA

The PLWHA belongs to the lower strata of the society with low or no levels of education attained. All the female PLWHA have been infected by their husbands through unprotected heterosexual intercourse and among men one has been infected through heterosexual intercourse and other three due to needle sharing. Majority of the women PLWHA were widows. Though they were widows and had to bear a lot of burden, they did not have any ill-feeling towards their husbands. They wished they were alive and sharing their pain. All the PLWHA are dependent on the few who have disclosed their status to the public and were working towards a viable environment where all the PLWHA could disclose their status and live without stigma and discrimination. They were concerned about the lack of comprehensive treatment at the Darjeeling District Hospital. Though all the PLWHA loathed the deplorable condition of the Darjeeling District Hospital and most of the staff, they only had words of praise for one lady doctor who was constantly at their service.

The main concern for the PLWHA was not only the absence of health facilities in Darjeeling but that they have to access NBMCH for any medical support they require. The fact that they face a lot of difficulties there due to language barrier and the attitude of the health workers makes them wary of going to NMBCH. Also the cost of travel is a major concern for them. The limitation of Darjeeling District Hospital to deal with the complexities of HIV/AIDS and the associated OIs was also a cause of worry for the PLWHA of Darjeeling hills.

The unavailability of ART was a reason for their apprehension about being able to lead a healthy life. Most of them related HIV/AIDS ultimately with death and sufferings. However, with the advent of ARVs this perception has changed over the period. With the advancement of medical science HIV/ AIDS is no longer equated with death and sufferings by the

PLWHA. The advent of ARVs and ART and the government's effort to provide it free of cost to the needy ones and also subsidize its cost has given hope to many. However, this hope and optimism depends largely on the state's sustained effort to provide free or subsidized ART.

The stigma and discrimination associated with the infection has become a hurdle for many to disclose their HIV sero positive status, even to their families. In such a social milieu few are willing to disclose their sero status. There are only five PLWHA who have disclosed their HIV sero positive status publicly. The PLWHA have to face discrimination in the health care settings. However, not much discrimination has been reported at the societal level. However, this is not an indicator towards a non-discriminatory environment as most of the positive individuals have not yet disclosed their status and the real social world will only be known when the society comes face to face with large number of people infected with HIV/AIDS. Though their life experiences have been bitter after being infected by HIV/AIDS they did not have any ill-feelings towards their possible infector.

The PLWHA felt that the community members did not have any knowledge about HIV/AIDS and that they perceived themselves to be out of the domain of the epidemic. They wished that community members would understand at the earliest that anybody can be infected by the virus. The PLWHA voiced dissatisfaction for lack of political will among the local leaders. According to them, the politicians were insensitive towards them and have not even shown any sign of effort to improve their situation.

Population Movement

Human mobility and person to person contact increases the chances of the epidemic spreading (Komatsu and Sawada 2007). Migration from Darjeeling hills has been the result of deplorable employment opportunities. There are recruiting agencies in Darjeeling hills which is facilitating migration and also word of mouth from friends of the opportunities outside is encouraging youth who are unemployed at their places of residence to migrate. One of the respondents said, *"When the youth working outside come home they encourage the others back home to migrate. At times they also arrange suitable unskilled jobs for their friends and siblings. In a situation like this, the boys at home feel useless when compared with those who have left their homes and gone out to work so they ask their friends to look for jobs. In my village there are hardly any youth these days."* Such migration can become a risk factor for the spread of HIV/AIDS as there will be absence of social support and network.

In the absence of social support and parental supervision and restriction young migrants indulge in risk behaviours. This makes them very vulnerable and susceptible to HIV/AIDS. Peer pressure among them also encourages them to take risk. In such a situation the young people in an endeavour to experience new things in life undertake risk behaviour as a form of entertainment. Due to ignorance of risk, lack of awareness and lack of access to health services these migrants expose themselves to HIV/AIDS. People go to nearby places like Siliguri, Kolkata and Kathmandu and avail the services of commercial sex workers. Many do not practice safe sex and expose themselves to STI/STD and HIV/AIDS. When they return, the people with whom they have sexual liaison like their wives, girlfriends and also the FSWs whose services they avail are put at risk due to their exposure outside.

Migrants easily find work in the informal sector. The low pay and the insecurity of job place them in an exploitative situation. They may face both sexual and economic exploitation at the hands of their employers and their companions. Women being alone look for companionship and intimacy. Their lack of education and awareness makes them vulnerable to sexual exploitation and thereby rendering them susceptible to a range of STI/STDs including HIV/AIDS. Those women who migrate to foreign countries also experience sexual exploitation by the employers and acquaintances.

The business communities who travel outside the hills also indulge in sexual activities with commercial sex workers in the places they visit for their business purpose. They have reported to have practiced unsafe sex. They may get infected during such exposure. They may transmit the virus acquired during such exposure to their partners and spouses with whom they have sexual relations. They are also susceptible to the danger of being infected with HIV/AIDS as they consume alcohol in the company of sex workers. As both the client and the service provider are in an intoxicated state they are in no position to take decision to protect themselves from the dangers of unsafe sexual practices and this renders them susceptible to HIV/AIDS and STI/STDs.

The greatest risk of HIV/AIDS through mobility is posed by the movement of the FSWs. The nature of their job warrants them to be on constant move. Their exposure to multiple clients elevates the chances of them getting infected, and thereby infecting their clients. They can spread the virus far and wide within a short span of time. Due to there low professional status and weaker bargaining position people do not pay any heed to the demands made by them for safe sex. The FSWs in such a situation for fear of losing their client seldom ask them to use condoms and this creates a conducive environment for the spread of HIV/AIDS. The risk taking irresponsible behaviour associated with movement of the people is a threat for the spread of HIV/AIDS rather than movement alone. Migration substantially increases the vulnerability of individuals to HIV infection, and also shapes the geographic distribution of the epidemic and the rate at which infection spreads. Thus, migration is both an individual risk factor as well as a structural factor driving the epidemic.

Sexual Behaviour

In this globalized world events in one part of the world has its impact on other parts as well. The changes in the sexual behaviour of the youth in Darjeeling hills are also influenced to a large extent by socio-economic and political developments around the world. The exposure the youth have had has encouraged them to become bold in every pursuit of life, and sex does not remain an exception. The youth are experimenting with sex and do not believe in sex being a taboo. Premarital sex which was rare even a decade ago has become common. Young boys are indulging in premarital sex under peer pressure to prove their masculinity. Girls are also seen engage in premarital sex for the experience of sex or to satisfy the demands made by their boyfriends.

It is not just premarital sex, but extra-marital sex was also found to be prevalent among respondents. The reasons for this are diverse. Extra-marital sex among the women is prevalent due to lack of attention by the husbands, to compensate for the low income in the family, and also to fulfil the needs generated by the emerging consumerist culture. Women's indulgence in extra-marital affairs can be attributed to factors like long absence of the husband, a kind of revenge for their husband's infidelity and desire for emotional support.

Unprotected heterosexual contact with multiple partners is the most common risk factor for HIV/AIDS associated with adolescents. There was lack of knowledge regarding safe sex and condom use. In such a situation if somebody is infected recently with HIV and does not know his positive status and indulges in unsafe sex then there will be a higher rate of HIV transmission.

More than 50 per cent of the male participants in the focus group discussion reported having multiple partners. The participants, especially males, in the study sample described widespread sexual and romantic networks, which were sustained by high levels of mobility and frequent movement in and outside the hills. Many married women and young girls with boyfriends have reported to be aware of their partner's other sexual relations. This places them within higher risk of getting infected by HIV/AIDS.

Fidelity practiced by only one partner does not necessarily provide enough protection from HIV/AIDS. In a situation where there is a significant proportion of the respondents engaged in sex with multiple partners HIV/AIDS can also infect the partner who is loyal in the relationship. In a scenario where there are many concurrent partnerships in the general population, then HIV/AIDS can become a generalized epidemic.

Condom Use

There are numerous evidences to prove the benefits of condom use during vaginal or anal sex. Despite this people still persist in having sex without condoms. This puts them in undesired risk of many sexually transmitted infections, including HIV/

AIDS and unwanted pregnancy. There are no particular groups who involve themselves in such risk, though sub-groups like the FSWs and IDUs indulge more in such risk. Irrespective of the socio-economic status or educational level people indulge in unsafe sex.

The awareness among the people regarding HIV/AIDS is low which is evident from the field data. The risk of HIV/AIDS is compounded by the fact that among the people the use of condom is low and sexual promiscuity is prevalent. Condom has still not caught the imagination of the people. People are not aware of the advantages of condom and still hold the preconceived notion that condom reduces the pleasure of sex. This inhibition among the people to use condom acts as an impediment for the control and prevention of HIV/AIDS. Condom is correlated with trust and fidelity and this also makes it difficult for the people, especially the women to discuss its usage. To a large extent condom can impede the sexual transmission of HIV/AIDS. However, its use is nominal among the respondents.

Men who use the services of sex workers will become the single-most powerful driving force in Darjeeling's HIV/AIDS epidemics. Since most of these men are married or have partners, significant numbers of 'low-risk' women who only have sex with their husbands/partners will be exposed to HIV/AIDS. Women are known to face dangers of STI/STD and HIV/AIDS within the institution of marriage but husbands do not encourage the use of condoms. Women cannot negotiate its use with their husbands as they are culturally trained to fulfil the demands made by their husbands. Culture demands women to be submissive in matters of sex so they cannot demand the use of condoms from their husbands and boyfriends. The issue of trust which is of paramount importance between couples also makes them vulnerable. Due to the trust they do not ask their husbands to use condoms while having sex. On the other hand, the fear of being questioned on their fidelity by the husbands also creates impediments for the women to ask their husbands to use condoms. Entrenched gender norms continue to constrain women's control over their sexual and reproductive lives and thereby make condom use infrequent during premarital and extra-marital sex and sex within marriage.

Married women constitute a group with distinct risk of HIV/AIDS and face a host of obstacles in making informed decisions in protecting themselves from infections. Women are less able to prevent exposure to HIV if they are uninformed and uncomfortable about seeking information, if they feel men make the decision and if they feel obliged to please men. Men may also be less able to use condom and more likely to be coercive if they believe that they are not able to control their sexual urges (Marin 1996). Marriage is an institution controlled largely by the family, though things are changing to a certain extent. Choice of a bride or and groom are still made by the family members. The family has a say in the reproductive activity of the couple. The pressure to bear a child and importantly to bear a son puts women under tremendous pressure to have unprotected sex which places them in constant danger of HIV/AIDS (Clark 2004).

Family Life Education

One of the most controversial issues in the history of the HIV/AIDS epidemic has involved the dissemination of HIV/AIDS related information to the public. In such circumstances family life education becomes imperative for the control and prevention of HIV/AIDS in the population. Those who were in favour of family life education, argue that it will protect people from making wrong decision regarding sex. It will help youngsters to protect themselves from unwanted pregnancies, STI/STDs and HIV/AIDS. Among those who disagree with it, there exists great fear that such programmes will cause the youth to become sexually more active which may as a consequence lead to an immoral social environment (Wierson and Bright 1996). They also say that since sex has become very common among the people of the hills, family life education will even encourage those who have abstained from it.

One of the problems of starting family life education programmes is that the teachers and the programme developers are not trained to carry out family life education programmes. The cultural values also act as an impediment to start such programmes. Even if such education is started in the Darjeeling hills the contents of the programme will be determined by the school boards and it may not be inclined to address the needs of the local community. Such programmes should target the girls as they are the most vulnerable and susceptible to HIV/AIDS. The programmes should focus on training the girls to negotiate safe sex. Other institutions implementing such programmes should also focus on girls as it is critical to target sexually active girls (FSWs and newly wedded wives) when teaching sexual negotiation skills and safe sex, as there is more likelihood that these girls will participate or will be forced to participate in unsafe sex by their husbands or their clients. The cultural practice of making the girls submissive to the demands of the boys makes it necessary for such education on sex to empower the girls to negotiate for safe sex and to reject any proposals for unsafe sex.

Communication Technology and HIV/AIDS

Mobile phones have revolutionized the communication technology. It has helped the world to come closer and be in touch however far one is from their near and dear ones. However, one of the results of using mobile phones is that it has helped to bring the FSWs closer to the community members. In a situation where there is no brothel for the sex workers to work from, mobiles have made it easy for the FSWs to carry out their business. The advent of mobiles has given a boost to sex industry and accessibility has increased in Darjeeling hills. Almost all the FSWs have reported conducting their business with the help of mobile phones.

From the fieldwork, it is evident that the mobiles have made it very easy and convenient for the FSWs of the hills to conduct their business. They are easily contacted by their clients even if they are not in the vicinity of the clients. Earlier as some of the FSWs have narrated it was difficult for them to search for clients as they had to stay at some place and there was also the danger of being ridiculed by the disgruntled clients. But today they are safe from such ridicule in public places as they can negotiate with their prospective clients on the phone itself. The FSWs also have more time in hand as they can be contacted by their clients wherever they are. With the help of the phones they are flying between places in short notices. They go to Siliguri only when they get calls and do not have to spent days looking for their clients as earlier.

It is not just the FSWs who have benefited from the use of phones but also the clients. At any point of time they can get in touch with the FSWs. It is easier for their clients to look for FSWs and as Darjeeling is a small place where anonymity is a rarity, the confidentiality of the client can be assured. Out of the 74 respondents who have reported using the services of FSWs, 69 have reported using their mobiles to avail the services of FSWs.

Alcohol and HIV/AIDS

The nexus between substance abuse and spread of HIV/AIDS is an established fact. Substance abuse often leads to loss of self-control which leads to deviant behaviour which are associated with high risk behaviours like multiple partners, and unprotected sex that places them at risk of contracting HIV/AIDS. The thought of sexual pleasure overrides the norms of safe sex in the intoxicated state. The young person due to their age and under the intoxication of alcohol practice unsafe sexual behaviours and thereby put themselves under tremendous danger of being infected by HIV/AIDS.

Alcohol consumption is widely found to correlate negatively with individual's condom use. This correlation could result from a proximate effect whereby drinking alcohol before having sex reduces the inclination to use a condom by lowering risk aversion. Individuals who drink frequently are more predisposed than those who do not to take risk. Thus, the correlation between drinking and condom use may stem from their joint association with risk taking orientation (Gerber and Berman 2008). The belief that consumption of alcohol also enhances the duration of sexual intercourse forces many to drink before sex and thereby reduce the odds of condom use and expose people to HIV/AIDS.

Alcohol consumption while it encourages risk behaviours also delays the health seeking behaviour among the people who consume it. Many of the alcoholics perceive their health problems to arise from their addiction and thus find remedy to their problems in abstaining from alcohol for a short period of time (Sundas 2004). In such a situation they may be diagnosed late for the virus and thus may be harmful for them.

FSWs and HIV/AIDS

To make an estimate regarding the number of FSWs in Darjeeling hills is difficult as they have been able to conceal their identity from the larger society. However, it is important to note that the sex works in Darjeeling are characterized by high degree of mobility. The FSWs are powerless in the power relation *vis-à-vis* their clients due to their low social as well as economic status. This renders them helpless in negotiating safe sex practices. They are also taken for granted by their clients as the FSWs are willing to do anything for monetary gains. This makes them open to sexual coercion, which further accentuates their vulnerability to HIV/AIDS.

The incidences of STD/STI among the FSWs are high and needs to be addressed to prevent the transmission of HIV. There is a danger of HIV being transmitted to one another as STI/STD is a recognized co-factor in the transmission of the HIV/AIDS.

The role of the sex trade is crucial in the spread of HIV/AIDS in Darjeeling hills. In Darjeeling, men who use the services of FSWs is far greater than IDUs and other at-risk groups, so this group of men are probably the most important 'determinant' of future rates of HIV. A high proportion of men in Darjeeling use the services of FSWs. The market for the FSWs is huge and such client turnover can become a major factor in the spread of HIV. Low levels of condom use during paid sex contribute to increasing HIV infection. Programmes for increasing use of condoms with sex workers will do more than any other intervention to control HIV infections in Darjeeling.

IDUs and HIV/AIDS

IDUs have been among the groups most affected by HIV/AIDS since the epidemic began. Sharing syringes is a very efficient way to transmit blood-borne viruses such as HIV, which can spread rapidly through the IDU population. The sharing of needles is thought to be more potent than sexual intercourse in the transmission of HIV (*www.avert.org*). There are numerous instances of high drug-related HIV sero-prevalence in the Darjeeling hills. Considering the extent of the drug abuse driven nature of the HIV epidemic in Darjeeling, there is a paucity of responses to drug demand reduction.

The sharing of contaminated needles and syringes among the IDUs of Darjeeling is the most potent cause for the spread of HIV/AIDS among them. The entire sample has reported sharing needles with their friends or fellow IDUs at the time of doing drugs.

Infected IDUs can introduce the virus into the sex trade in two ways: as buyers and as sellers (female drug injectors). Female injectors are known to sell sex for drugs and significantly less likely to use condoms. This will lead to a very fast growth and spread of HIV/AIDS. The presence of multiple partners of the IDUs and the irresponsible sexual behaviour is a cause of concern for every authority engaged in the control and prevention of HIV/AIDS. They have reported to have used the services of the FSWs and not to have used condoms. This combination of the IDUs and the FSWs is very potent in the spread of HIV/AIDS. The personal perception of the IDUs about their life also adds to the danger of the spread of HIV/AIDS as they do not consider themselves to be productive and useful to the society and thus continue with their deviant lifestyles. Though IDUs have more knowledge about HIV/AIDS among the at-risk population their relation with the society *vis-à-vis* the status they are ascribed has to an extent been responsible for their irresponsible behaviour.

Bisexuals and HIV/AIDS

The use of alcohol and drugs and the absence of condom use among them is the greatest threat their behaviour poses for them. Because of their hidden nature it is very difficult to educate them regarding safe sex practices. Being close knit they have multiple partners among themselves and this along with the fact that they do not use condom exposes them to the risk of HIV/AIDS infection. Since their number is small and they are seen as deviants they are ridiculed by the society so the bonding within the group is very strong which makes it difficult for them to refuse sexual advances made by others. They predominantly prefer men over women for sex but due to taboo on same sex and societal pressure they also have sex with women to disguise their orientation. This places the women at risk of contracting HIV/AIDS.

Knowledge and Perception of HIV/AIDS among the People of Darjeeling Hills

Even after decades of awareness campaign, the awareness and knowledge about HIV/AIDS among the people is dismal and is directly proportional to education (Thimothy and Rajan 2004) and the many youth who are vulnerable to it are not well aware of sexuality, sexual health and HIV/AIDS as their sources of information are incorrect and unreliable (Acharya 2008). The people of Darjeeling hills were not well aware of HIV/AIDS. Only a few knew all the modes of transmission and some even reported that kissing can transmit the virus. Misconception regarding HIV/AIDS was found among some of the respondents and accurate knowledge about it was also missing. In addition to misconceptions about HIV transmission, many adults also hold misconceptions about HIV prevention and treatment. Almost every respondent had heard about HIV/AIDS. However, knowledge of many was limited to just the word 'HIV/AIDS'.

The backbone of HIV/AIDS control and prevention VCCTC was known to even fewer respondents. Out of the 199 respondents who were asked whether they had heard about VCCTC in the district an overwhelming 136 respondents denied having heard about the VCCTC. There were only 10 respondents who had ever visited the VCCTC. Only 1.5 per cent women had visited the VCCTC.

The respondents were not aware that HIV/AIDS is a consequence of many structural factors and it is determined by the socio-economic and political condition of the people. They thought that it was solely a medical issue. However, many respondents were aware that there is no cure for the infection but were not aware that there were medicines to prolong the life of the PLWHA. Regarding the concept of 'ABC', respondents were not aware of it. Knowledge of HIV/AIDS was very limited among the people which are also a danger for the proliferation of HIV/AIDS cases in the hills of Darjeeling. Knowledge about HIV/AIDS can prevent from acquiring the virus but was blatantly missing among the people.

Stigma and Discrimination in the Darjeeling Hills

The greatest impediment to prevent the spread of HIV/AIDS is the stigma and discrimination associated with it. Stigma and discrimination also hinders providing adequate care, support and treatment. Stigma and discrimination associated with HIV/AIDS is universal, occurring in every region of the world. They are triggered by many forces, including lack of correct understanding of the disease, lack of treatment and the fact that it is incurable.

There are evidences of the existence of stigma and discrimination in Darjeeling hills. However, the frequency and intensity of this is much lower than in many parts of the country as most of the PLWHA have still not disclosed their HIV sero positive status. HIV/AIDS related stigma and discrimination undermine Darjeeling's responses to the epidemic, preventing people from using a range of important services. Discrimination against PLWHA affects their access to employment, education and importantly health, Strong prejudice against PLWHA has been found in health services. Furthermore, those groups that are most at risk of HIV/AIDS infection are already discriminated against, stigmatized and marginalized.

Discrimination at the familial level has also been reported. At this level the women are the victims. There has been an instance where the in-laws have chased away their daughter-in-law after their son died of AIDS. The fact that many of the PLWHA have not disclosed their positive status to their family also suggests that there is the fear of being discriminated by the family. Even in the employment sector there has been discrimination for the PLWHA.

There is a high degree of acceptance among the high risk group for those infected by the virus. Among the high risk group the IDUs showed greater acceptance followed by the bisexuals and the FSWs respectively. This can be due to the fact that they perceive themselves to be at risk.

HIV/AIDS related stigma poses a problem for all in the society thereby imposing severe hardships on the people who are its targets and it ultimately interferes with treatment and prevention of HIV infection. Emphasis on the eradication of HIV/AIDS related stigma would enable in creating a social climate conducive to a rational, effective and compassionate response to the epidemic.

Experiences of PLWHA and the Care Givers

All the PLWHA were acutely aware of the thought that came to their mind when asked to get tested for HIV/AIDS. They were initially offended by even the mere suggestion to get tested. Respondents though they had heard about HIV/AIDS they themselves never perceived it as something that would affect or infect them.

The males who actively pursued sharing of needle or had sex with multiple partners never seem to have been aware of the dangers of HIV/AIDS. This lack of awareness created a sense of invulnerability. So when they tested positive for HIV/AIDS it is understandable that it must have been a moment of utter shock and disbelief. The first thought for most of the respondents was to think that the test results were incorrect or that the hospital staff had mixed up their blood sample for someone else's. As their only knowledge of HIV/AIDS was that it was an incurable disease leading to quick death, they were overcome with the feeling of utter desperation. Many were suicidal and worried about their parents and families as to how they would cope up once the PLWHA were gone. The PLWHA were guilt ridden for what they perceived as having brought about untold misery to their loved ones. Strangely none of the PLWHA showed any anger or animosity towards their infectors. The wives seem to have forgiven their husbands, most of whom had died. The IDUs too felt no anger as they realized now that there was no awareness about HIV/AIDS. They by and large felt that there must be many more cases among other IDUs who have not got themselves tested. Once they tested positive, they were advised by the doctors not to disclose their HIV sero positive status. The doctors probably feared that the PLWHA would face discrimination and stigma which would only aggravate matters. The PLWHA too don't want to go public with their positive status. As a result only 5 PLWHA have come out in the open. By and large the rest remain hidden from what they see as a hostile society. As they face discrimination and ill-behaviour at the hospital itself, their fear is justified. When health officials who are supposed to be in the know-how about the disease exhibit prejudices, one can only gauge what the response of the lesser informed public can be. The PLWHA do not only go through emotional trauma but also suffer from financial constraints. Lack of proper medical facilities at their place of residence meant they have to travel longer distances to avail health facilities.

The care givers also wanted to keep the identity of their wards a secret. They feared stigma and discrimination against the entire family. For most of the care givers the topmost priority was to increase the life span of their loved ones. But many were also concerned about higher economic costs of looking after a PLWHA especially after the onset of full blown AIDS.

Institutional Response to HIV/AIDS in the Darjeeling Hills

After the onset of HIV/AIDS the international community came forward to challenge the virus which has been termed as the greatest killer in human history. International agencies such as the UN, WHO, UNICEF etc. have worked in their own way to stop the epidemic from doing further damage to the human society. Likewise the national governments have also contributed towards the prevention and control of the virus. The Indian Government responded to the threat of HIV/AIDS by constituting NACO and implementing the national programme to control and prevent the virus.

Even after the concerted efforts by the Indian Government, the virus has entered different regions and has moved away from the identified risk population to the community members. Darjeeling has lately experienced the impact of the virus. There have been institutional responses to control and prevent the virus from affecting more people but it has not been effective and sufficient. At the forefront has been Shanker Foundation.

It tries to address the concerns of the positive people with its limited financial as well as human resources. The foundation has been reaching out to other people with HIV/AIDS with very little means of support. The challenge of constant care and support to the increasing number of people living with the disease is a daunting task for the foundation. There is a lack of technical help and the positive members themselves have to work in addressing these issues which it considers to be pressing and important. Among the many issues it is the social stigma and discrimination that they face which is considered the most daunting.

Shanker Foundation, like the population it serves often finds itself in a position of vulnerability. It is most vulnerable to the withdrawal of support from the DACC and other institutions that have been offering them help and support till now. While it has achieved a strong profile in its field and can count on help from the many well-wishers, the overall tolerance and support for its work is volatile.

The single most important strength of Shanker Foundation has been its ability to improve the quality of life of its members. However, there are other indicators that show success of a different kind. An important indictor has been the Foundation's ability to attract volunteers who do not have a direct stake in HIV/AIDS. For instance, in addition to the PLWHA and their relatives, the Foundation has attracted the participation of a number of volunteers who are not HIV sero positive and have no family members living with the virus.

Other than Shanker Foundation there are many NGOs working in the field of HIV/AIDS. They are supporting the PLWHA and also disseminating knowledge of HIV/AIDS to the public. However, the dissemination of knowledge has to be more vigorous as there are still many who have not heard of it or have inaccurate knowledge. There are many NGOs working in Darjeeling hills in the area of HIV/AIDS education, control and prevention but the models of these programmes are drawn from NACO, which draws heavily from the western model of HIV/AIDS prevention and control and lack utterly the much required understanding the local dynamics of the epidemic. The strategies employed by these NGOs are also based on the guidelines and recommendations of NACO. The result is an emphasis on awareness building and portrays HIV/AIDS as an infectious and a fatal disease associated with the deviants such as the intravenous drug users and commercial sex workers. The awareness building campaign, led by various NGOs have been fairly successful at promoting this association with HIV/AIDS in the Darjeeling hills. Such an association has in fact, lead many to believe that they are safe from HIV infection.

The lack of research and theoretical framework has made it very difficult for the NGOs to achieve desired results. Apart from this, there is no data collected by the individual NGO of the population they are working with. Even the minimal data collected by some of the NGOs are not shared with others. Though all the NGOs are linked with the DACC and Shanker Foundation, this link is tenuous. There is a lack of proper coordination among the NGOs. Increased collaboration could facilitate the development of a common language to describe approaches so that practitioners can better understand one another's work. Although some networking does occur through the DACC, the experience in conducting this study has shown that the networking among the different organizations could be significantly improved. Through discussions conducted during the course of the study, it was established that various NGOs were not familiar with the work of other organizations. In spite of this, there are glimpses of efforts being made to improve on networking among the different organizations.

DACC is the only funding agency for the NGOs working in the Darjeeling hills and also acts as a bridge between the NGOs, the community and the government and is under tremendous pressure to perform. However, the government has failed to understand this which is reflected by the fact that the DACC is understaffed. Because of the lack of staff the DACC has not been able to generate commitment and sense of urgency among the people and the disbursement of funds to the NGOs has also been slow. This has in turn had a negative impact on the functioning of the NGOs immensely.

As mentioned earlier apart from DACC there is no involvement of other agencies including the two giant players—the tea industry and the railways. The people of Darjeeling are serving both these sectors since its inception. In return they have not shown any commitment towards the HIV/AIDS menace in Darjeeling hills. The DACC must pressure them to engage in the ongoing battle against HIV/AIDS.

The NGOs also report that as the DACC is the sole funding agency it tends to fund only programmes which have been carried out elsewhere and which it sees as safe. This method has not borne any fruit as is seen in the prejudices and half-baked knowledge about HIV/AIDS among the community members.

In the Darjeeling hills there is a real danger that the prospect of an epidemic will attract individuals and organizations whose interest will lie solely on the resources that are now being increasingly made available to the NGOs for work on HIV/AIDS related issues and will not serve the interest of those who are directly and indirectly affected by the disease. There are NGOs which are discarding their earlier programmes and are working with a certain high risk group which they think will provide them more funds and that they can therefore work for a longer period of time rather than scaling up their existing programme.

The educational, political and medical institutions are not very engaged in the control and prevention of HIV/AIDS. Many of the schools do not have any programmes building awareness of HIV/AIDS among its students. The government in order to educate the students about HIV/AIDS has initiated the School AIDS Education Programme and is being implemented in many schools across the nation. However, this programme is not implemented in the hills of Darjeeling primarily as the schools are reluctant to initiate this programme and they also lack the resources to start such programme, in terms of trained personnels to start such programme.

In Darjeeling apart from MANAS Bangla there are no other institutions which focus on MSM. The communication tools of these organizations only focus on the transmission of HIV/AIDS through heterosexual mode thereby shifting the overall focus from the dangers posed by anal and oral sex, which are common among the highly vulnerable group such as the homosexuals. The language of the campaigns in Darjeeling is also not clear and ambiguous phrases are used such as safe sex, sexual intercourse and sexual contact and fail to impart the correct information to the layman. They shy away from using appropriate terms such as semen, vaginal fluids, oral and anal sex etc. which would give a clearer picture of HIV/AIDS and its modes of transmission. The programmes addressing HIV/AIDS issues among MSM and bisexuals are left largely to MANAS Bangla. Therefore, each and every organization working in the area of HIV/AIDS must reach out to the MSM and address the needs of this group.

The political leaders are at a vantage point for disseminating information on HIV/AIDS as their reach is broader and wider. The political parties are not showing any inclination to involve themselves with issues related to HIV/AIDS. They largely view it as a health issue which the health department should be concerned with. The frequent bandhs which are being called in the renewed demand for Gorkhaland is also hampering the PLWHA's accessibility to the much needed medical facilities.

The VCCTC was started in Eden Hospital on the 1st of April, 2002. Various behavioural change communication initiatives were undertaken targeting those who indulge in high risk behaviour. Testing, counselling, prevention of parent to child transmission and post-prophylaxis is provided here. However, for CD4 cell counting and ART, the PLWHA have to go to NBMCH, Siliguri. The VCCTC is located at the basement of the hospital so its visibility is low. Also the PLWHA reported that the health staff showed insensitivity and did not respect the need of the PLWHA for confidentiality. Apart from this VCCTC, there are no other testing centres in the study area which spreads over 1421.54 sq.kms. Coupled with economic deprivation and poor infrastructure facilities, the conditions of the PLWHA remains grave. It is important to note that a VCCTC opened at Kurseong had to be closed as the hospital could not provide it with any space to function.

Overall, the response to HIV/AIDS in the Darjeeling hills has not been very productive if one looks at the very low levels of awareness regarding the disease. The involvement of *'samajs'*[1], which has a greater larger reach than the NGOs is absent. In an endeavour to concentrate on the prevention of HIV/AIDS most of the NGOs and other institutions have overlooked the basic forms of dissemination of information like the IEC material which are more attractive and also provides privacy to the individuals who read them to learn about HIV/AIDS.

For example HIV/AIDS related posters in English and Nepali were not seen anywhere. There were no posters and festoons regarding the transmission, risk factors, symptoms of HIV/AIDS and the myths regarding HIV/AIDS. The only one at Kurseong Hospital was covered with moss. Brochures and informational materials were not frequently distributed by the NGOs in the Darjeeling hills.

All the institutions in the Darjeeling hills have to come together to prevent and control the further onslaught of HIV/AIDS. It also becomes mandatory for them to engage the PLWHA in the formation and implementation of the programmes. The NGOs should also look for the mandate of the community in their work and should also focus their work on the rural population who has been ignored till now. The NGOs are not working independently on the issue of stigma and discrimination which is one of the most salient barriers to the control and prevention of HIV/AIDS. There is not much effective response to the HIV/AIDS related stigma and discrimination in the Darjeeling hills. For this the NGOs have to work simultaneously on several fronts, like awareness building, sensitization and capacity building of the PLWHA as well as other vulnerable groups.

Findings

Knowledge of HIV/AIDS

HIV/AIDS has been found to be associated with a large number of socio-economic factors which are central to the smooth functioning of our daily life. However, the widely held view is that it is a medical issue and people from Darjeeling hills do not take into account the associated socio-economic variables into consideration. For them it is merely a medical issue. 66.33 per cent people reported it to be a medical issue.

Complete and correct knowledge about HIV/AIDS is considered to be the first and foremost requisite to save oneself against this fatal disease. Only a few respondents knew all the four modes of transmission. All the respondents knew that HIV/

AIDS is transmitted from human to human but only 12 (6.03%) respondents (excluding the PLWHA) knew all the 4 major routes of transmission. A total of 13 respondents have reported that HIV spreads through kissing. Women lack knowledge of the modes of transmission of HIV/AIDS.

The concept of 'ABC' was the initial step to control the spread of HIV/AIDS and subsequently which became the pillar on which the prevention and control of the epidemic worldwide rests upon is still not known to many in the hills. The total number of people who have heard about this concept is 21. Among these 21, only 4 are female and none of the females who fall in the risk category have reported to have known about 'ABC.'

That there is a VCCTC in Darjeeling is known to only 31.65 per cent of the respondents. The percentage of people unaware of the presence of VCCTC in the district is very high at 68.33 per cent. Along with the low level of awareness, the people also have many misconceptions regarding HIV/AIDS. Apart from the community members, even the level of understanding and awareness among the health care personnel is low, incorrect and incomplete. Breast feeding was not thought to be a mode of transmission, even by some of the health staff.

Sexual Behaviour and Safe Sex Practices

Sexual behaviour has gone a sea change over the years. The myth about sex has been broken and it no longer holds to its sacrosanct nature. It has been experienced, experimented and debated. The people of the hills due to the heterogenetic and orthogenetic changes taking place in the society have started to change their perspectives regarding sex. These changes in the attitude of the people regarding sex, especially among the youth, have led to increase in casual premarital sex. This has become a danger for the further acceleration in the rate of HIV transmission among the people of the hills as casual sex is on the rise, safe sex practices are non-existent.

Findings from the fieldwork data revealed that at the time of the first sexual intercourse none of the respondents perceived themselves to be at risk of HIV. For most of them pregnancy and not sexually transmitted infections were of primary concern. The analysis of the context of the first sexual intercourse reveals that young people in general and male youth in particular, were highly motivated to have sex because of the social and cultural expectations to prove their manhood, to identify with their peers and to satisfy their sexual needs or curiosity. Therefore, the motivations for the first sexual experience seemed to override any concerns of HIV risk.

The study finds that the youth in the hills have a very early sexual debut and premarital and extra-marital sex among both the male and female informants is relatively common. 68.34 per cent respondents reported having premarital sex and 22.61 per cent respondents reported extra-marital sex. The percentage of respondents reporting multiple partners was 62.81 per cent. 45.22 per cent of the respondents were sexually active while travelling. It can be deciphered that they use the services of the CSWs when travelling and this can translate into a very quick transmission of HIV among the people. This practice of indulging in sex while travelling is not confined to the males alone but even the female respondents have reported to have engaged themselves in sexual activities while being away from home. 16 female respondents have reported to have engaged themselves in sex while travelling. Indulging in sex while away from home has been a satisfying experience for many women. The primary reason for many to indulge in sex while travelling was the sexual gratification they experienced, which their husbands could not provide. These women could not engage in sexual partnership more openly and regularly at their home towns as they were aware that being a small place their escapades could at anytime become public which would bring disrepute to themselves. In the 15-20 age group, 12 out of the 30 have reported to have had had sexual exposure. Many of them have reported to have had sex in Siliguri with CSWs. This is a disturbing trend as their eagerness to experience sex may prohibit them from practicing safe sex and thereby exposing them to the dangers of HIV/AIDS.

Culture of a place and community is largely responsible for the sexual behaviour of its people. The culture of Darjeeling does not permit the females to be sexually active or informed. This leads to the low use of condoms and more importantly females are handicapped by the culture to demand their partners to use condoms while having sex or to learn about sex and transmit the knowledge to their male partners. The practice of safe sex and the use of condoms are relatively low among the respondents. Among the community members only 21 respondents reported using condom, while none of the FSWs and the IDUs reported using condom. Only 2 women have reported using condom. Out of the 9 bisexuals in the sample, only 3 reported condom use. There are only 24 respondents who have reported using condom. Though people have multiple partners and are using the services of FSWs, the use of condom is minimal. There is a negligible per cent of both the male (4.02%) and female (2.51%) respondents who speak about HIV/AIDS while discussing sex and even fewer discussing condoms among the female (1.50%) respondents. Condom is discussed only as a means to prevent pregnancy and not as a protection against STI/STD and HIV/AIDS. The female respondents did not have any control over the issue of condom use even within marriage and this poses a danger as many male respondents have reported to be indulged in extra-marital sex, used the services of FSWs and CSWs. The female respondents did not see themselves being in a position to negotiate safe sex.

Multiple partners among the sample population are very much evident and this is a great concern in the hills of Darjeeling. As men and women have multiple partners in addition to their husbands, wives and partners, long-term parallel sexual partnership will be a very important dimension in the spread of HIV/AIDS in the hills of Darjeeling. It has been recognized that the men who migrate are a risk to the community as they are exposed to the virus when engaged in sexual relations with CSWs when their wives are not around. However, in the hills it is evident that the wives are also engaging in sexual relations with other people when their husbands are not around and may act as a vector to pass on the virus to their husbands.

Stigma and Discrimination

Across the world, the global pandemic of HIV/AIDS has shown itself capable of triggering responses of compassion, solidarity and support, bringing out the best in the people, their families and communities. But the disease is also associated with stigma and discrimination, as individuals affected or believed to be affected by HIV have been rejected by their families, their loved ones and their communities. This rejection holds true in every part of the globe. All-over the world, ignorance, lack of knowledge, fear and denial have engendered serious and often tragic consequences, denying PLWHA access to treatments, services and support, as well as making it hard for prevention work to take place.

As in other parts of the world stigma and discrimination was found to be prevalent in the hills of Darjeeling. The PLWHA in the sample reported to have been discriminated at some point of time. Discrimination has been reported from the hospital, at the familial level and while giving employment. This discriminating attitude of the people has stopped the PLWHA from disclosing their positive status. The lowest rate of discrimination was found within the risk groups.

The health care staff also feared discrimination for the PLWHA and encouraged them not to disclose their sero status. Consequently, the PLWHA did not disclose their status and reported that it gave them a sense of great relief and strength.

Intravenous Drug Users

Only as late as 2002, the first case of HIV/AIDS was confirmed in the hills of Darjeeling. There were many youth who had started using drugs out of peer pressure, desperation and lack of other creative avenues. The drug users and especially the IDUs were and are an isolated group who share needles and syringes in their isolated dens. Most of them do not know that HIV could be transmitted through blood and sharing of needles.

Today there are almost 1200 drug abusers registered with the Red Cross Society alone and the hidden population of the drug dependents can still be very high. The sexual behaviour of the IDUs in the hills of Darjeeling is also irresponsible as one of the doctors have narrated. Among the IDUs, the presence of multiple sexual partners is also common. The IDUs though inducted in some of the awareness programmes behave in irresponsible manner when they are intoxicated. This irresponsible behaviour is a cause of worry among many who work to control and prevent the spread of HIV/AIDS in the hills of Darjeeling. More importantly the IDUs do not perceive themselves to be of any use to the society. This forces them to be irresponsible and care much for their welfare of the self and the other, which becomes dangerous for the prevention and control of HIV/AIDS.

People Living with HIV/AIDS

All the PLWHA were either infected heterosexually or by sharing of needles. All the women PLWHA whether married or not were infected by their husbands or their partners. The widows were being looked after by members of their family of origin or natal. The PLWHA felt that others will see them as immoral people and so will shun them. Some of the PLWHA married or single had aspirations of raising a family but the disease has created doom and hopelessness as all of them knew that regardless of the ART available there was no permanent cure for the infection.

The female PLWHA did not have any ill-feelings against the person who infected them. At times of depression and desperation they thought about their partners and wished that they were alive. The widows wished their husbands were alive for the social support they would provide at times of need. They in tune with the tradition revered the departed souls and had no ill-feelings towards them, though they knew that they were infected by them.

The burden of the disease was perpetually being faced by the women as they were left to look after the children after the death of their husbands. There were 6 widows (31.6%) among the 19 ever married female members of Shanker Foundation. This is relatively a high figure in the initial stages of the epidemic. The burden of the disease is severe for them as they are not educated and also do not have any formal vocational training to secure a livelihood.

Flying Sex Workers

The FSWs are a constant threat to the spread of the HIV/AIDS as they are not just confined to the hills but work in other places as well. Their low bargaining power and the use of alcohol makes it difficult for them to negotiate safe sexual practices. They along with their clients do not use condoms. The level of awareness regarding HIV/AIDS among them also acted as an obstacle for them to insist on condom use. Their reach which is much larger than those CSWs stationed at brothels also poses a greater threat for the spread of HIV/AIDS in the hills.

Responses

The early response to HIV/AIDS in the hills of Darjeeling was the establishment of the VCCTC. However, the VCCTC was only set up at the district hospital and this has restricted the reach of VCCTC to a large extent. The people especially of the rural area have not been able to utilize the facilities provided by the VCCTC. The VCCTC has shrugged off its responsibility and sends all those who are found to be positive to Shanker Foundation for further counselling, care, treatment and support though post-exposure counselling is part of their responsibility.

The other lines of response are the NGOs which are linked to the DACC and Shanker Foundation. However, the collaboration between them is very weak. They only fulfil their professional needs rather than collaborate and work for the emancipation and betterment of the PLWHA. The programmes carried by the NGOs are high risk group centric and the need to sensitize the community members is not understood by the programme implementers. The programmes are targeted interventions and the community members are left out. The NGOs have not made any effort to engage the railways and tea gardens in the fight against the infection. Further the tea gardens and the railways have not voluntarily come forward to confront the disease.

The governmental and non-governmental organizations have directed efforts to improve policies and programmes to meet the needs for sexual health information and services of the young people and thereby reduce the incidence of HIV/AIDS. However, the progress to reduce their sexual risks has been slow and these efforts have not had any significant consequences in the lives of the people. Knowledge about the sexual behaviours of the people and the factors influencing these behaviours in Darjeeling hills is unreliable and lack of data has prevented attainment of a deeper understanding of the determinants of safer sexual practices which is necessary for the development of effective interventions.

Strategies for Confronting HIV/AIDS in Darjeeling

The hills of Darjeeling saw a quick response to the HIV/AIDS epidemic and the DACC was established for its control and prevention. As it has become evident that the epidemic is not just a bio-medical problem there is a dire need to confront the disease in a more holistic manner. The reasons for the spread of the disease in different parts of the country are diverse so planners need to implement programmes that keep local differences in mind. To effectively control and prevent the virus from further spreading in the region there is a need to put in place a locally viable programme and strategies which are conducive to the local environment and is culturally acceptable.

For any major programme to be successfully introduced and sustained, participation of all sections of the society is a requisite. This is especially true when one is dealing with a disease like HIV/AIDS. Compartmentalized efforts like the targeted interventions, lectures in schools, flyers and posters pasted at certain points will not bear much result. As HIV/AIDS is a result of a combination of social, economic, political and medical factors all these aspects have to be borne in mind. HIV/AIDS also involves personal issues like sexual habits and preferences so to target these various issues a sensitive, holistic model has to be created. Figure 6.1 gives the diagrammatical description of the strategy that could be implemented in Darjeeling hills for effective control and prevention of HIV/AIDS epidemic.

As NACO and WBSAC&PS are the nodal agencies at the national and the state level their participation is also needed to provide training and expertise to the NGO staff, other health service providers and the local administrators. Health service providers from the grass root level have to be inducted in this. After the training, the responsibility of the NGO activists is to train the community members like the school teachers, *panchayat* members, members of caste *samajs*, members of clubs

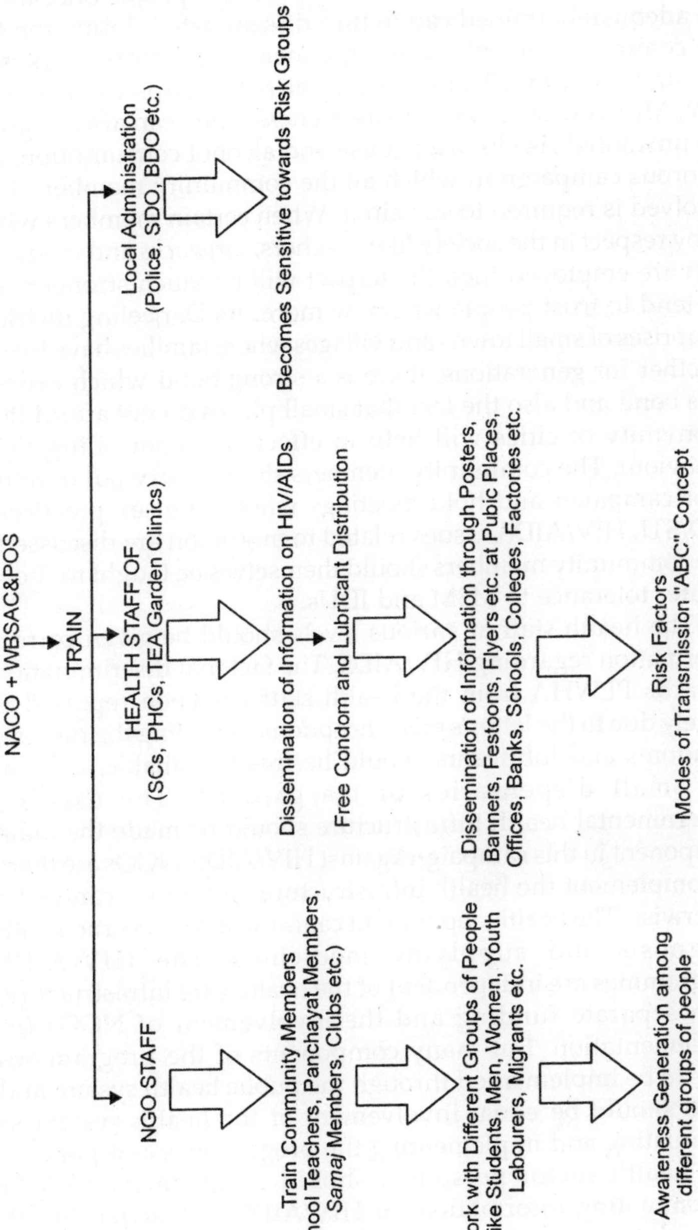

Fig. 6.2: Depiction of Model Strategy to Control and Prevent HIV/AIDS in Darjeeling Hills

etc. through seminars and workshops. These people once they are adequately trained can in turn disseminate information to the community members at large including factory workers, labourers, migrant labourers and at-risk groups to generate HIV/AIDS and sexual health awareness. They can also control the unwanted rise in drug abuse and alcohol consumption. A vigorous campaign in which all the community members are involved is required to sustain it. When certain members who enjoy respect in the society like, teachers, *sarpanchs* and medical staff are employed then the impact will be much stronger, as we tend to trust people we know more. As Darjeeling district comprises of small towns and villages where families have lived together for generations, there is a strong bond which exists. This bond and also the fact that small places do not afford the anonymity of cities will help in effectively controlling risk behaviour. The community members should carry out door to door campaign and hold meetings where safe sex practices, STD/STI, HIV/AIDS, issues related to migration are discussed. The community members should themselves be taught to show greater tolerance to MSM and IDUs.

The health staff at various levels should be given correct information regarding HIV/AIDS. The fact that discrimination towards PLWHA from the health staff has been reported is largely due to the latter's misconceptions regarding the disease. Condoms and lubricants should be freely available, even in the small dispensaries of tea gardens. The existing governmental health infrastructure should be made the main component in this campaign against HIV/AIDS. NGOs are there to complement the health infrastructure and things cannot be otherwise. The health department cannot just be concerned with diagnosis and supplying medicines. The HIV/AIDS programmes are independent of the health care infrastructure, with separate funding and the involvement of NGOs for implementation. But many components of the programmes have to be implemented through the public health system and there should be equal involvement of the health system in formulating and implementing the programmes and policies. The health sector personnel should be given the task of disseminating information on HIV/AIDS and sexual health through the use of posters, flyers, banners and festoons at important public places, offices, banks, schools, club houses and hotels.

Regarding the administration, the police, BDOs, SDOs should all be sensitized about the issue of HIV/AIDS. As and when they come across IDUs, MSM, FSWs and alcoholics, the police should send them to the NGOs or community groups who can teach these high risk groups aspects of leading a healthier life. The local administration should provide logistic help to other parties. There should be interdependence and coordination among these groups.

To control the spread of HIV/AIDS in hills, an effective strategy at the district level must be built to control and prevent it. Under the tripartite agreement between the Central Government, State Government and the GNLF, the DGHC was formed. The Health Department came under its purview. DGHC due to many reasons has been ineffective in developing a proper health infrastructure in the region. Now the advent of HIV/AIDS is infecting and affecting a large number of the population, the State Government cannot afford to leave the onus of providing adequate health facility to a non-functioning DGHC alone.

The State Government must render all possible help required for controlling and preventing the spread of HIV/AIDs and also make the concerned authorities accountable. The State Government should monitor the functioning of DACC. As the DACC functions under the aegis of DGHC, the State Government has to pressurize the Member Secretary of the DACC to become proactive and not confine himself to just signing the cheques. DACC has to undertake capacity building measures for its staff as they are responsible for formulating and implementing programmes on HIV/AIDS in the hills. The DACC has to advocate for making the NBMCH accountable for all the difficulties faced by the PLWHA from the hills while visiting it. DACC must focus in formulating programmes which address the needs of the local population and should not just implement policies and programmes formulated by NACO or WBSAC&PS. It should involve Shanker Foundation and other NGOs in formulating programmes. As it is the bridge between the people and the elected representatives of DGHC, it needs to be active to convince them about the importance of their participation and thereby develop a political will against HIV/AIDS. DACC should not be constrained by the bureaucratic protocols and should be as transparent as possible. It has to make its reports accessible to all. They should encourage researches and researchers and should not let the protocols be a barrier to such collaborations.

NGOs are a powerful weapon in the fight against HIV/AIDS. They have to be well versed with the developments taking in the field of HIV/AIDS in Darjeeling as well as outside. They should document information regarding the epidemic in a more professional manner and share information amongst themselves. Their existing programmes must be upgraded instead of changing them in anticipation of greater fund from the funding agencies. As was evident in the course of the fieldwork, the manpower in many of the NGOs were not qualified to carry out the task in hand. Therefore, the NGOs should make every possible effort to impart different trainings to their staff whenever possible and also focus on capacity building of their staff.

NGOs in Darjeeling hills were found to be more urban area centric. Focus needs to be given to rural areas as well where information on HIV/AIDS is abysmally low. Informing such deprived areas in time can help a lot. More importantly many from the tea gardens are migrating and due to their low educational level and lack of information do not know the intricacies of HIV/AIDS and thus become vulnerable. They should undertake interdisciplinary studies on their own to understand the local dynamics of the epidemic. NGOs should share the findings of such studies amongst themselves so that it becomes easier for all to tackle the epidemic. They should network and collaborate with each other in understanding the issues of social development, gender equity and social exclusion, which can help them formulate programmes to fight stigma and discrimination.

Some of the public sector enterprises such as Steel Authority of India (SAIL), Indian Railways and Employees State Insurance Scheme (ESIS) have associated with NACO in controlling the disease through various ways. NGOs in the hills have to encourage the railways as well as the tea industry to collaborate with them to control and prevent the spread of HIV/AIDS. Tea companies under the corporate responsibility can be asked to supply ARV drugs required for HIV/AIDS affected poor people in the tea gardens.

NGOs play a vital role in changing the risk behaviour of the risk groups. They have to encourage the members of the risk groups to come forward and gather information on the epidemic. They have to provide the support these groups require and gain their confidence so that they can work with them more effectively and efficiently. After gaining their confidence they should work towards sensitizing them about the risk involved in their behaviours. NGOs have to impart knowledge about STI/STD and HIV/AIDS to them so that they become aware of the risk they are taking and can also consciously try to change their behaviour patterns. As most of the FSWs have at some point of time been infected with STIs they have to make aware that STIs and STDs are recognized factors of HIV/AIDS. Free condoms should be made available to the FSWs and they must be encouraged to use them. NGOs also have to make arrangements for medical support to the risk groups as they may be reluctant to visit the health service providers. The NGOs should try to create an incentive structure that will assure an adequate level of participation by the members of the target population.

The hospitals and the health service providers have to support the NGOs in this regard. The district health department should collaborate with the NGOs in building awareness through campaigns on sexual health for both men and women, addressing the problems of RTI/STI and its linkage with HIV/AIDS. In doing so they should also encourage the people to use condoms. They have to undertake STI/STD, HIV/AIDS surveillance among the risk groups and migrant labourers who come to Darjeeling hills. The treatment seeking behaviour of the risk groups should be encouraged. Community members and bridge population like the drivers have to be encouraged to participate in the awareness building campaigns and prevention programmes. The focus of the prevention programmes should be the use of condoms as it is a recognized barrier against HIV/AIDS. To successfully encourage condom use among the people regardless of sub- group, gender or risk category there has to be a high level of social support in improving the negotiating power and skill of the female partners. As there are many who migrate to other places, NGOs should collaborate with the recruiting agencies which send people out to impart knowledge about safe sex, condom uses, RTI/STI/STD and HIV/AIDS.

The health authorities as well as the NGOs in collaboration with educational, religious institutions have to undertake studies to understand the sexual behaviours of the people. This will in turn help them formulate and implement policies and programmes which will encourage people to change their sexual behaviour and practices. This will also help the NGOs in identifying the gaps of the programmes they are implementing at the moment. The successful design and implementation of such programmes will ultimately improve the welfare of the youth. The foundation of such programmes must be accurate information about their sexual and risk taking behaviour and the unyielding understanding of the underlying dynamics.

IDUs are the most infected group in the hills. They must be encouraged to seek medical as well as psycho-social help. NGOs should work towards educating the parents of the IDUs regarding their conditions. Parents should be taught that the IDUs require medical intervention as well as social support. IDUs should not be frowned upon rather they should be encouraged to participate in the NSEP and OST programmes. IDUs should also be made aware of their irresponsible sexual behaviour and encouraged to use condoms. They should be encouraged to feel a part of the society and that they are equally responsible for the functioning of the society.

Over the counter sale of drugs is very common in the hills. It is very important for the NGOs to convince the chemists not to sale drugs without prescriptions from doctors. Strong police action have to undertaken against these defaulters. The NGOs should also conduct orientation programmes with the chemists and make them realize the contribution they can make to eradicate drug addiction by not selling drugs to people who come without prescription.

The police department should also be sensitized regarding the sensitivity of drug addicts and addiction. They should be encouraged to tackle this problem in a more humanitarian way rather than enforcing the law and arresting them. There should be collaborations between the police department and the NGOs, especially the IRCS so that if the police come across any drug dependent person they refer them to IRCS for NSEP or OST. Recreational facilities should be made available for the youth as they have high energy level which needs to be properly channelized. In the absence of such facilities many youths are indulging in drug abuse due to boredom.

The involvement of *samajs* in the control and prevention of HIV/AIDS in the hills should be made mandatory by the concerned authorities. The *samajs* exercise so much social control over its members that they can make a lot of difference by their participation as they have direct contact with the members. The decisions taken are by and large binding upon the members, so they can have immediate impact on the prevention and control of HIV/AIDS. The participation of the *samajs* in HIV/AIDS prevention and control programmes also means the participation of larger number of people whether directly or indirectly.

There is not much effective response to the HIV/AIDS related stigma and discrimination in the hills of Darjeeling. For this the NGOs, government institutions, media all have to work simultaneously on several fronts, like awareness building, sensitization and capacity building of the PLWHA as well as other vulnerable groups. The involvement and the participation of the *samajs* can also reduce the stigma and discrimination against the PLWHA. The involvement of *samajs* means the involvement of the community members so once they are involved stigma and discrimination can be brought down.

Dissemination of information has been the backbone of raising awareness among the community members. Every tool and technique should be experimented to disseminate information regarding HIV/AIDS in the hills. Public display of banners, posters and festoon are the primary mode to disseminate information to the public. Not much effort was evident on the part of the authorities to inform the community members through this mode. Therefore, it becomes imperative to display such information at public places and places where there is likelihood of people gathering. The letters and information should be very visible, graphic and attractively written. The language used should be very simple and easy to comprehend. Care should be taken that such banners and posters should not be obstructed by anything.

Another important means of disseminating information about HIV/AIDS in the hills is the involvement of clubs, especially the football clubs. As the people in the hills are football lovers, clubs can be utilized to disseminate information about HIV/AIDS. Pamphlets can be distributed before the match starts and even the clubs can be asked to organize awareness campaigns for their supporters.

Educational institutions are known to make the future citizens of a country. Their responsibility lies in producing well-groomed and well-informed citizens. However, today the most important information for everybody has inevitably been the information on HIV/AIDS. These institutions have to impart information on HIV/AIDS to their students. The participation of the educational institutions in the hills was found to be lax. Therefore, they must be involved in the dissemination of knowledge about HIV/AIDS. They should not leave it up to the NGOs to come to the schools and provide information on HIV/AIDS to the students.

Educational institutions should be encouraged to encourage their wards to gain knowledge about sexual health and teachers should be trained to impart such knowledge to their pupils in a scientific and interesting manner. They should also encourage parents to participate in such activities as the involvement of the parents will enhance the effectiveness of such endeavours. Schools and colleges should take the onus of encouraging parents to talk about sex and HIV/AIDS with their children. They should also make a conscious effort to implement standardized educational programmes on HIV/AIDS.

As most of the people in the hills use mobile phones it can be used to disseminate knowledge about HIV/AIDS. Mobile service providers should be encouraged to disseminate knowledge about HIV/AIDS. Messages related to HIV/AIDS awareness should be sent across population on regular basis and not just once every year, on 'World's AIDS Day.' The NGOs working with the vulnerable groups can also make use mobiles to encourage them to use condoms and at times of difficulties provide the help they need. When the FSWs are with their clients, NGOs can with the collaboration of the FSWs disseminate information on the benefits of condom use.

Notes

1. *Samajs* are community based organizations and in the Darjeeling hills it is caste based. All the families belonging to a caste has to become a member of its *samaj*.

Chapter VII

Summary and Conclusion: Will HIV/AIDS Triumph Over Mankind in Darjeeling?

Summary of the Thesis

Ever since the first case of HIV/AIDS was detected in June 1981, in the United States of America, the disease has managed to grab headlines the world over. Having caught the public imagination, responses to it both at the national and international levels have been spontaneous. Especially when we compare it to other life threatening diseases like malaria, tuberculosis or even more 'mundane' issues like death due to hunger. There have been many programmes funded by the many institutions. Various international and national NGOs and even private foundations like the Bill and Melinda Gates Foundation have devoted time and poured huge amount of funds to fight this incurable disease. World leaders of the G8 nations have pledged unstinted support and initiatives like 'Treat 3 Million by 2005' have been implemented. There has been no lack of will in combating HIV/AIDS. However, the question that remains unresolved is that in spite of all the efforts that seems to have been put in, why is there still a rise in the number of infections annually? The virus has long moved from being a "gay disease" and affecting those indulging in high risk behaviour to seemingly low risk groups.

HIV/AIDS is making huge inroads from the vulnerable urban areas to fairly cocooned small towns and villages. Before the 5 PLWHA publicly disclosed their HIV sero positive status in May 2007, in a local daily the community members of Darjeeling hills had probably never in their wildest imagination conceived of the virus reaching Darjeeling hills. HIV/AIDS was and still is seen as a disease which is "somewhere out there" in the West or at the margins of society, far away from the average man and woman. So what has led to the rise in the number of HIV/AIDS infected individuals in Darjeeling? What factors have contributed to its spread? What have been the institutional responses? What are awareness levels among the community members, the at-risk groups such as FSWs, IDUs and bisexuals and the health personnel? What are the probable strategies to confront HIV/AIDS in Darjeeling? These and other related issues have been dealt with in this book.

The first case of HIV/AIDS in Darjeeling hills was detected in 2002 in an IDU after the only VCCTC was set up in Darjeeling District Hospital. As mentioned earlier this number rose to 141 by November 2007. However, it is important to note here that there is only one VCCTC for the entire Darjeeling hills which covers an area of 1421.54 sq. km (area of the study area). Lack of proper roads, low levels of education, economic deprivation and low level of awareness about HIV/AIDs make the only VCCTC in the area inaccessible to the majority of the population who reside in remote villages and tea gardens. It can safely be stated that if the number of surveillance centres are increased then these numbers will also multiply.

A socio-political and economic overview of Darjeeling hills will make it evident as to why the area is so conducive to HIV/AIDS. Politically Darjeeling has been highly volatile for the last three decades. Demands for separation from West Bengal in the early 1980s, led to political unrest where many lost their lives in 'police encounters' and 'custody.' Finally in 1987, the Darjeeling Gorkha Hill Council was formed. The demand for the separation which centred on issues of identity, unemployment, lack of infrastructure and development were not resolved even under the DGHC. The funds that were granted by the state were misused by the political leaders. Economic opportunities remained low and frustration levels high. Casualisation of jobs led to the youth being further disgruntled. Drug abuse and alcohol consumption rose as a consequence.

Tea gardens and railways are the two major employers in Darjeeling hills. However, increasing lack of job in the railways has led to economic insecurities. Globally the expensive Darjeeling tea is facing stiff competition from Sri Lanka, China and Kenya forcing many tea gardens to close down. Even where the tea gardens are still functioning, the income levels of the workers remain low and many are not on the permanent payroll. Most are employed as casual labourers during the plucking season. There are harrowing instances where mothers give rice beer, a homemade alcoholic beverage from left over rice to infants to tide over hunger pangs (Sundas 2004).

The quality of education is very poor and economic levels are very low and this in turn is forcing many to migrate. These migrants are devoid of any social network which forces them to indulge in risk behaviours which subsequently intensify their vulnerability to HIV/AIDS. Many women migrate to share the burden of the family. Due to their low education level and absence of any vocational training they find jobs in the informal sectors and mainly work as domestic helps. They are vulnerable to various kinds of exploitation. Many seek companionship and sometimes are deceived into prostitutions in the promise of better jobs.

In the urban area many youth are attracted to the metros for jobs in the BPOs. Away from home and societal restrictions and the availability of disposable cash pushes many to involve in casual sex and other risk behaviours. Many are found to indulge in drugs and alcohol. Those joining the army are also known for their risk taking behaviour which may make them susceptible and vulnerable to HIV/AIDS. These people act as vector and may transmit the infection they acquire to the people back home.

A number of people from the hills have been joining the army. HIV/AIDS cases have been detected among the army personnel as they avail the services of CSWs, so there is a possibility that when they visit home they can act as vectors.

The belief that condom use lowers sexual pleasure is the main reasons for the very low use of condom and thereby proliferate the individual's risks against STI/STD and HIV/AIDS. The FSWs, who are constantly engaged in sexual activities with a large number of clients also do not insist on condom use. Their social status and lack of any power within the relationship with the client also renders them powerless to negotiate condom use and safe sex practices. It has also been reported by both the FSWs and their clients that they consume alcohol before sex. In their inebriated state safe sex and condom use does not even cross their minds.

The reach of the FSWs is very wide, in terms of the spatial distribution of their clients as well as their movement. In such a circumstance they can act as a vector to a large number of people distributed across different regions. They are not just confined to the hills of Darjeeling but travel outside Darjeeling to conduct their business. This further aggravates the situation. As there is no brothel based sex industry in Darjeeling hills, the identity of the FSWs remain hidden so targeted intervention among them remains a major challenge. There has been manifold increase in the business of FSWs with the introduction of mobile phones. Mobile phones are being successfully used to increase their reach to clients. The anonymity which the phones provide makes it easier for the clients to avail their services too without the danger of being exposed in public. Earlier it would had been much more difficult to proposition a sex worker.

Other changes have also been noticed in the society. Attitudes of the youth towards sex are also changing very rapidly. This can be attributed to the changes that are taking place at the global level. The youth are indulging in casual premarital sex. Sex is no longer seen as a private act between married couples. The respondents have also shown indulgence in sex with multiple partners. Many married respondents have also reported to have indulged in extra-marital sex which is against the traditional norms and values. None however, seems to see condom use as necessity. It was primarily seen as a technological invention to prevent pregnancy. Multiple partners and unsafe sex can render one vulnerable to HIV/AIDS. Such irresponsible behaviour among the husbands has placed their wives at a risk of HIV/AIDS infection. It was also seen while conducting the research that married women had no say in condom use. Another important reason for not using condom has been the overemphasis or trust and love by the wives on their husbands.

As noted earlier, the first case of HIV/AIDS in Darjeeling was detected in an IDU. Drug abuse has been prevalent in Darjeeling hills since the 1980s which coincided with the demand for a separate state. Punk culture also influenced many to do drugs which they saw as hip. Drug addiction is a grave problem in Darjeeling hills. Drugs are easily procured from either the porous Nepal border or from the North East states. However, there has not been any institutional response in dealing with this problem. As seen in the study carried out by the researcher awareness levels regarding HIV/AIDS is very low. Some were found to know about HIV/AIDS being transmitted through needle and syringe sharing but mostly saw them as being relatively safer. They also indulged in sex with other IDUs and FSWs which further aggravates the situation. In their desperation for a *'fix'* the IDUs do not care much about safe injecting practices. Many of them are also married which places their spouses at risk.

Alcohol is an integral part to the culture of the hills. However, alcohol use has been on the rise and increasingly young high school boys and girls have started consuming alcohol. Alcohol consumption is related to risk behaviour. Also alcohol consumption has an adverse impact on the health of the people. It has been found that most of the people use alcohol to get rid of the inhibition they have regarding sex. Under the influence of alcohol it is difficult for them to practice safe sex thereby making both the partners vulnerable to STI/STD and HIV/AIDS.

Darjeeling has been identified as most vulnerable to HIV/AIDS by NACO and WBSAC&PS. As seen earlier factors conducive to the spread of HIV/AIDS places the community members at a great risk *vis-à-vis* HIV/AIDS the community members showed ignorance about the epidemic. It may be because of this that the PLWHA do not want to disclose their status as they fear prejudices, stigma and discrimination from the public. What is grave is that even the hospital staff also exhibits such prejudices against the PLWHA and do not show them any empathy. This has created a major hindrance among the PLWHA to seek whatever little facilities the hospitals provide. They prefer to avail the services of the NGOs instead.

In Darjeeling the main actors involved in combating HIV/AIDS are the DACC, Shanker Foundation and a number of NGOs like the Sewa Karya, MANAS Bangla, HANDS etc. DACC provides the various organizations with the required funds, Shanker Foundation is the only network of positive people in Darjeeling hills and other NGOs are working in the field of HIV/AIDS and other related issues. Much needs to be done in terms of generating more funds and collaboration between various organizations. Shanker Foundation is doing enormous work among the PLWHA but there is a paucity of funds as well as lack of human resources to carry out sustained advocacy. Most of the PLWHA have not disclosed their sero status so the work of the entire organization rests upon few shoulders.

Tea gardens and railways have shown utter lack of corporate responsibility towards the control and prevention of HIV/AIDS in Darjeeling hills. Political leaders view it as health concern so have washed their hands off it completely. The DGHC is functioning without any political participation since its dissolution in 2002. So no political pressure can be exerted and no one in the higher echelons of the administration seems to be concerned about this issue.

There is an immediate need to upgrade health facilities including surveillance centres, ART centre and the availability of ARV and other facilities such as CD4 cell counting, hospice, care and treatment. Dissemination of information on safe sex has to be prioritized by the authorities.

Summary of the Findings

The primary mode of transmission of HIV/AIDS in the hills of Darjeeling is injecting drug use and heterosexual intercourse. The knowledge about HIV/AIDS among the sample population was very negligible. Though they knew that it could be transmitted during sexual intercourse they were not aware of the other modes of transmission. It was not just the community members who were lacking in the knowledge about the epidemic also many in the health sector did not know all the 4 modes of transmission of HIV/AIDS. The concept of ABC which has been successful in controlling and preventing the spread of HIV/AIDS was also not known to many.

Sexual behaviour of the sample population, whether at risk or not, was fraught will danger of getting infected. There is a widespread prevalence of premarital and extra-marital sex among them. The use of condom is minimum among the MSM, IDUs and FSWs do not use them. Young boys are buying sex to prove their masculinity or simply out of curiosity regarding sex. Alcohol consumption among the FSWs and their clients is high which also reduces the practice of safe sex. There are about 1200 registered IDUs in the hills of Darjeeling. Apart from sharing needles the presence of multiple partners heightens the spread of HIV/AIDS in Darjeeling hills.

The mobility of the IDUs, FSWs and the behaviour of the community members when away from home also increases the risk of HIV/AIDS transmission. FSWs because of their mobility can spread the virus far and wide. The community members may be exposed to the virus while using the services of the commercial sex workers.

There are 141 cases of HIV/AIDS reported in the hills of Darjeeling and the number is presumed to be just a tip of an iceberg. The response to the epidemic was found to be lax. The DACC which is the most important institution for the control and prevention of HIV/AIDS in the hills is caught up in the bureaucratic protocol and has not been able to generate any political will to fight the dreaded virus. The NGOs are also not fully equipped to control and prevent the epidemic from further spreading. There is very little collaboration among the various NGOs working in the area of HIV/AIDS in Darjeeling. The dissemination of information among them was found to be negligible though efforts are being made to improve networking. The involvement of railways and tea industry is also negligible though they have a large section of the population as its employees.

PLWHAs of the hills find themselves to be helpless whenever they have to visit NBMCH. Their experiences show that they have had bitter experiences at the hospitals and at the hands of the health care-providers. They longed for the support of their partners at the times of distress and difficulties and they did not have any ill-feelings towards the person who may have possibly infected them.

Summary of the Strategies

A broad but inclusive strategy is required to combat the disease. All members of the society, health personnel, police, NGOs, administration of all levels must be engaged in this task. Information dissemination is key to fighting this disease and public participation is crucial to carry out a sustained campaign. Door to door campaign, free condom, information on safe sex is vital in this regard. Strategy at the district level is necessary for the control and prevention of the virus. The State Government should also be active and not leave the onus of controlling HIV/AIDS in the district to the DACC alone and not leave it as independent vertical programme. The control and prevention of HIV/AIDS should be made a part of the overall health programme. The DACC which is the nodal agency for controlling HIV/AIDS in the hills of Darjeeling should be made more accountable and proactive. It should advocate with NBMCH for providing better facilities to the PLWHAs from the hills.

NGOs have to be more active in the rural areas as these areas are out of the ambit of control and prevention programmes. The focus of the NGOs should change from urban areas to tea gardens from where there are many youth migrating to other places. NGOs have to collaborate among themselves and share the information they have about HIV/AIDS in the hills. NGOs have to work hand in glove with the *samajs* as they can effectively help in the participation of larger number of people. Their reach is also greater and can directly or indirectly help the information and messages reach its members.

NGOs have to also engage the at-risk groups and encourage them to participate in prevention programmes and in their targeted intervention campaigns. They should be encouraged to adopt safe sex practices. They should be empowered to negotiate safe sex and condom use with their clients. Incentives should be provided to all those at risk group people who participate in the programmes and also arrangements have to be made for them to undergo tests for STI/STD and HIV/AIDS.

The chemists should be sensitized to the dangers posed by selling drugs over the counter without the prescription of doctors. They should be made equal partners in the control of drug addictions which may also help in the reduction of new HIV/AIDS infection. The police department should also be made partners in the control of drug addiction. They should be sensitized about the behaviours of IDUs and other drug dependent persons. They should be asked to deal with the drug dependent persons with empathy rather than implementing the laws which can be harsh. They should be made aware that these people are like any one of the community members and with proper care and handling can give up the habit of drug abuse.

Educational institutions should take the responsibility of educating its students regarding HIV/AIDS and dangers posed by drug abuse. Teachers should be involved and schools and colleges should not rely too much on the NGOs for providing such information to the students. Parents and guardians of the students have to be made part of such programmes in the schools and colleges.

Conclusion: HIV/AIDS and Human Security in Darjeeling

The aspect of human security is very important while dealing with HIV/AIDS in Darjeeling. Though the impact of HIV/AIDS in Darjeeling has not been severe enough to warrant a study of human security but it will not take much time for such a study to be a necessity. People here in Darjeeling are facing insecurity in terms of decreasing agricultural land, rapidly decreasing job opportunities and lack of proper health infrastructure. HIV/AIDS has a severe impact on food security, affecting all of its dimensions: availability, stability, access, utilization. One of the most devastating impacts of the AIDS epidemic is the loss of human capital, as the disease robs households of adult labour and knowledge. The agricultural sector (including the tea industry) in Darjeeling will be under a particularly severe strain as the HIV/AIDS epidemic spreads, affecting and infecting more people. Given its effects on agricultural production and other livelihood strategies, HIV/AIDS will lead to a reduction of the amount of food available to individuals, households and communities. As the agricultural sector is a labour intensive sector, the health of the youth is of paramount salience and their inability to work will impact the production which will directly and indirectly have an impact on the lives of thousand of individuals. This may lead to lower food intake, thus reducing both individual nutritional status and household food security.

The people of the hills are also insecure about their employment. As already mentioned in the earlier chapter, many people engaged in tea industry are employed as casual labourers and some only during the plucking season, so they don't have a steady source of income. There is a constant threat to their well-being and consequently many migrate to other parts of the country and expose themselves to the risk of HIV/AIDS. Apart from the insecure nature of employment in the tea industry, jobs in other sectors have also witnessed rapid casualisation. After the formation of DGHC in 1989, the employment scenario has not improved but has in fact further deteriorated. The State Government has virtually stopped recruiting people in the hills and recruitment is only on daily wage basis. This casualisation of labour in Darjeeling has made the people very insecure in terms of employment and their economic condition.

Prevalence of HIV/AIDS is determined by the policies and magnitude of development. Its severity is associated with various dimensions of poverty. Poverty not only increases the chances of HIV transmission, it also increases the sufferings of PLWHA. In the wake of globalisation, the present model of development promotes rapid migration from rural to urban areas. Migration from Darjeeling is also facilitating the growth of HIV/AIDS cases in the hills. Many of the female PLWHAs reported to be infected by their husbands who were working in cities.

With the growing number of HIV/AIDS cases, safe sexual practices, safe injecting practices and responsible individual behaviour is important to check the transmission of HIV. Among the people of Darjeeling responsible behaviour, with their sexual partners, including FSWs is essential to control the spread of epidemic. Ensuring individual responsible behaviour is difficult if other spheres of the society do not reflect responsibility in their intent and content. Along with the individual social responsibilities, there is need for other domains also to show responsibility towards society. State should be responsible towards the well-being of the people. Health system should reflect concerns towards providing universal access and affordable healthcare services. Also doctors should show commitments towards the patients. Community should reflect on the socialisation processes and societal values, and also be responsible for its members (Ritu Priya 2003).

As stated in the hypothesis, poor socio-economic conditions and lack of infrastructure is pushing people towards risk behaviour and making them vulnerable to HIV/AIDS. This statement is seen to hold true for the hills of Darjeeling.

For the community to triumph over HIV/AIDS it becomes imperative for every body to be responsible towards each other. Being responsible reduces alienation, stigma and discrimination of those infected by the virus and thereby lessens the burden of the PLWHAs. Being responsible and involved reduces the fear of HIV/AIDS among the community members, which is responsible for stigma and discrimination. When such a situation arises where there is no social alienation, stigma and discrimination and people as well as the state and other spheres of society fulfils their social responsibility will human triumph over HIV/AIDS.

Bibliography

Bhat, R. and Saha, S. (2004), "Financing Issues in Proposed HIV/ AIDS Interventions of Providing Antiretroviral Drugs to Selected regions in India", IIM, Ahmedabad, May.

BMJ Editorial (1996), "Caring for patients with HIV and AIDS in middle income countries", BMJ Editorial, British Medical Journal, Volume 313, No. 7055, August 24.

Family Health International, (2004), "Attitudes and Beliefs Towards People Living with HIV/AIDS—Nepal", Kathmandu, Nepal.

NACO (2007), "NACP-III: To Halt and Reverse the HIV/AIDS Epidemic in India", *http://www.nacoonline.org/upload/Publication/IEC%20&%20Mainstreaming/NACP%20III%20-%20To%20Halt%20and%20Reverse%20the%20HIV%20Epidemic%20in%20India.pdf*, retrieved on 25.03.08.

PANOS, (2000), "Comparative analysis: Research studies from India and Uganda".

"Access to Treatment: The Cost of Treating HIV/AIDS in India and Nepal", *http://www.panossouthasia.org* retrived on 23.4.06.

"HIV awareness tops minister list", *The Telegraph*, Siliguri, April 8, *http://www.darjeelingtimes.com/news/News/India-not-ready-to-legalise-commercial-sex.html*, retrieved on 9.4.2008.

"HIV Prevention, Harm Reduction and Injecting Drug Use", *www.avert.org*, retrieved on 7.6.2006.

Acharya, S., (2008), *Health and Sexuality Among Youth in Uttarakhand (India)*", Man-Development, Vol. 30, No. 3, pp. 71-86.

Action Aid, (2006), *Positive Voices: Emerging Governance Issues on HIV and AIDS in Asia*, Shivam Sundaram, New Delhi.

Aggleton, P., (2001), "Gender and HIV/AIDS: What Do Men Have To Do With It?", *Current Sociology*, Vol. 49, No. 6, November, pp. 23-37.

Ainsworth, M. and Teokul, W., (2000), "Breaking the Silence: Setting Realistic Priorities for AIDS Control in Less-Developed Countries", *The Lancet*, Vol. 356, pp. 55-60.

Altman, D., (1999), "Globalisation, Political Economy and HIV/AIDS", *Theory and Society*, Vol. 28, pp. 559-584.

Amathya, S., (2005), "Gender and HIV/AIDS in Nepal: Some Observations", *Indian Anthropologist*, Vol. 35, No. 1-2, March/September, pp. 139-152.

Amin, A. (2004), ''Risk, Morality and Blame: A Critical Analysis of Government and US Donor Responses to HIV Infections Among Sex Workers in India", Centre for Health and Gender Equity, *http://www.wfsnews.org/ngoreports.ph p?db=wfs&table =NGOReports&mediasection=Reports%20/%20Books&page=3*

Ankrah, E.M., (1991), "AIDS and the Social Side of Health", *Social Science and Medicine*, Vol. 32, No. 9, pp. 967-980.

APN+, (2004), "AIDS Discrimination in Asia", *http://www.gnpplus.net/regions/files/AIDS-asia.pdf* retrieved on 5.4.2006.

APN+., (2004), "AIDS Related Discrimination and Human Rights", *http://www.ahrn.net/library_upload/uploadfile/file1778.pdf* retrieved on 4.3.2005.

Arunkumar, T.S. *et al.* (2004), "HIV Patients: Knowledge and Sexual Behaviour Patterns", *EPW*, Vol. 39, No. 12, 20-26 March, pp. 1208-1210.

Ateka, G.K. and Selwyn, B.J., (2007), "Adolescent Human Immunodeficiency Virus and Sexually Transmitted Disease Prevention Programmes: Are Gender-Blind Approaches Justified?" *Public Health*, Volume 121, No. 9, September, pp. 682-689.

Bagla, P., (2007), "India's New HIV/AIDS Number", *EPW*, Vol. 42, No. 30, 28 July-3 August, pp. 3080-3081.

Barnett, T., (2004), "AIDS in India: Disaster in the Making", *EPW*, Vol. 39, No. 39, 8-14 May, pp. 1888-1892.

Berkman, L.F., & Kawachi, I., ed, (2000), *Social Epidemiology*, Oxford University Press, New York.

Bharat, S., and *et al.*, (2001), "India: HIV and AIDS Related Discrimination, Stigmatisation and Denial", Geneva, Switzerland, UNAIDS, *http://data.unaids.org/Publications/IRC-*

pub02/JC587-India_en.pdf retrieved on 7 *Studies in family Planning*.6.2006.

Bhat, R. and Shah, S., (2004), "Health Insurance: Not a Panacea", *EPW*, Aug 14.

Blance, A.K., (2001), "The Effect of Power in Sexual Relations on Sexual and Reproductive Health: An Examination of the Evidence", Vol. 32, No. 3, pp. 189-213.

Bor, R, & Elford, J. ed, (1996), *"The Family and HIV"*, Cassell, New York.

Brinkhof, M. WG *et al*., (2008), "Early Loss of HIV Infected Patients on Potent Antiretroviral Therapy Programmes in Lower Income Countries", *Bulletin of the WHO*, Vol. 86, No. 7, pp. 559-567.

Burtney, E. and Duffy, M. ed (2004), *"Young People and Sexual Health: Individual, Social and Policy Contexts"*, Palgrave, New York.

Campaign for Access to Essential Medicines, (2005), "Amendment to WTO TRIPS Agreement Makes Access to Affordable Medicines Even More Bleak", 7 December, *www. www.accessmed-msf.org/prod/publication.asp?scntid=* 71220051425522&contenttype=Para&. retrieved on 7.11.2006.

Campbell, C.A., (1991), "Prostitution, AIDS, and Preventive Health Behaviour", *Social Science and Medicine,* Vol. 32, No. 12, pp. 1367-1378.

Carballo, M., & Siem, H., (2002), "Migration, Migration Policy and AIDS" in Haour-Knipe & Rector (ed), *Crossing Borders: Migration, Ethnicity and AIDS,* Taylor & Francis e-Library, London, *www. gigapedia.org,* retrieved on 4.9.2007.

Catalan, J., Sherr, L., & Hedge, B., (2005), ed, "The Impact of AIDS: Psychological and Social Aspects of HIV Infection", Taylor & Francis e-Library, Amsterdam, *www. gigapedia*.org, retrieved on 4.9.2007.

Chimbiri, A.M., (2007), "The Condom is an 'Intruder' in Marriage: Evidence from Rural Malawi", *Social Science & Medicine,* Vol. 64, No. 5, March, pp. 1102-1115.

Clarke, S., (2004), "Early Marriage and HIV risks in Sub-Saharan Africa", *Studies in Family Planning,* Vol. 35, No. 3, pp. 149-160.

Collins, J. and Rau, B., (2000), "AIDS in the Context of Development", Social Policy and Development Programme Paper No. 4, December, United Nations Research Institute for Social Development, *http://www.unrisd.org* retrieved on 26.2.2006.

Cooper, D., Harries, J., *et al.* (2007), "Life is Still Going On": Reproductive Intentions Among HIV-Positive Women and Men in South Africa", *Social Science & Medicine*, Vol. 65, No. 2, July, pp. 274-283.

Cornman, D.H. *et al.* (2007), "An Information-Motivation-Behavioural Skills (IMB) Model-Based HIV Intervention For Truck Drivers In India", *Social Science & Medicine*, Vol. 64, No. 8, April, pp. 1549-1559.

Craddock, S., (2007), "Market Incentives, Human Lives and AIDS Vaccines", *Social Science & Medicine*, Vol. 64, No. 5, March, pp. 1572-1584.

Cunningham, I., *et al.* (2005), "Ten Years of AIDS Images in the Puerto Rican Press: 1983-1992", in Catalan, J., Sherr, L., & Hedge, B., (ed), "The Impact of AIDS: Psychological and Social Aspects of HIV Infection", Taylor & Francis e-Library, Amsterdam, *www. gigapedia.org*, retrieved on 4.9.2007.

Dasgupta, A., (1999), "Ethnic Problems and Movements for Autonomy in Darjeeling", *Social Scientist*, Vol. 27, No. 11/12, Nov-Dec, pp. 47-68.

Dash, A.J. (1967), "Bengal District Gazetteers: Darjeeling", Bengal Government Press, Alipore.

D'Cruz, P., (2004), *Family Care in HIV/AIDS: Exploring Lived Experience*, Sage Publications, New Delhi.

Deacon, H. & Boulle, A., (2007), "Commentary: Factors Affecting HIV/AIDS-Related Stigma and Discrimination by Medical Professionals", *International Journal of Epidemiology*, Vol. 36, No. 1, Feb, pp. 185-186.

DeJong, J., (2003), *Making an Impact in HIV and AIDS: NGO Experiences of Scaling Up*, ITDG Publishing, London.

Delhi AIDS Control Society., (2005), *HIV/AIDS in Delhi: Meeting the Challenges.*

Deng, R., Li, J., Sringernyuang, L., Zhang, K., (2007), "Drug Abuse, HIV/AIDS and Stigmatisation in a Dai Community in Yunnan, China", *Social Science & Medicine*, Vol. 64, No. 8.

De Waal, A. and Whiteside, A., (2003), New Variant Famine: AIDS and Food Crisis in Southern Africa, *The Lancet*, Vol. 362 No. 9391, pp. 1234-1237.

Diamond, C., and Buskin, S. (2000). "Continued risky behaviour in HIV-infected youth", *American Journal of Public Health*, Vol. 90, pp. 115-118.

District Statistical Hand Book, Darjeeling, 2001.

Dodoo, F. Nii-Amoo, Zulu, E.M., Ezeh, A. (2007), "Urban-Rural Differences in the socio-economic Deprivation—Sexual Behaviour in Kenya", *Social Science & Medicine*, Vol. 64, No. 5, pp. 1019-1031.

Dunkle, K.L., Rackel, K.J., Brown, H.C., *et al.*, (2004a), "Gender-Based Violence, Relationship Power and Risk of HIV Infection in Women Attending Antenatal Clinics in South Africa", *The Lancet*, Vol. 363, No. 9419, pp. 1415-1421.

——, (2004b), "Transactional Sex among Women in Seweto, South Africa: Prevalence, Risk factors and Association with HIV Infection", *Social Science & Medicine*, Vol. 59, No. 2, pp. 1581-1592.

Dunkle, K.L., Rackel, J., Mzikazi, N., *et al.*, (2007), "Transnational Sex with Casual and Main Partners among Young South African Men in Rural Eastern Cape: Prevalence, Predictors, and Association with Gender-Based Violence", *Social Science & Medicine*, Vol. 65, No. 6, pp. 1235-1248.

Eaton, L., Alan, J.F., Leif, E.A., (2003), "Unsafe Sexual Behaviour in South African Youth", *Social Science & Medicine*, Vol. 56, No. 1, pp. 149-165.

El-Bassel, N., White, S.S., Gilbert, L., Wu, E., Chang, M., Hill, J., and Steinglass, P. (2003). "The Efficacy of a Relationship-based HIV/STD Prevention Programme for Heterosexual Couples", *American Journal of Public Health*, Vol. 93, No. 6, pp. 963-969.

FHI, (2004), *Stigma & Discrimination Study in Nepal: Community Attitudes and the Forms and Consequences for People Living with HIV/AIDS*, Kathmandu, Nepal.

Fidler, R.D., (2004), *SARS, Government and the Globalization of Disease*, Palgrave, New York.

Ford, N., and Koetsawang, S., (1991), "The Socio-Cultural Context of the Transmission of HIV in Thailand", *Social Science and Medicine*, Vol. 33, No. 4, pp. 405-414.

Friedman, S.R., *et al.*, (2005), Network and Socio-historical Approaches to the HIV Epidemic among Drug Injectors", in Catalan, J., Sherr, L., & Hedge, B., (ed), *The Impact of AIDS: Psychological and Social Aspects of HIV Infection*, Taylor & Francis e-Library, Amsterdam, *www.gigapedia.org*, retrieved on 4.9.2007.

Gadd, K., & Goss, D., (2005), "HIV/AIDS Education in the Workplace: It's Not My Responsibility..." in Catalan, J., Sherr,

L., & Hedge, B., (ed), *The Impact of AIDS: Psychological and Social Aspects of HIV Infection* Taylor & Francis e-Library, Amsterdam, *www. gigapedia.org*, retrieved on 4.9.2007.

Gatrell, C.J., (2007), "Secrets and Lies": Breastfeeding and Professional Paid Work", *Social Science & Medicine*, Vol. 65, No. 2, pp. 393-404.

Gerber, T.P., & Berman, D., (2008), "Heterogeneous Condom Use in Contemporary Russia", *Studies in Family Planning*, Vol. 39, No. 1, pp. 1-17.

Godbole, S. & Mahendale, S. (2005), "HIV/AIDS epidemic in India: Risk Factors, Risk Behaviour and Strategies for Prevention and Control", *Indian Journal of Medical Research*, Vol. 121, pp. 356-368.

Goode, W.J. and Hatt, P.K. (1987), *Methods in Social Research*, McGraw-Hill Book Company, Singapore.

Gregson S., Nyamukapa, C.A., Garnett, G.P., *et al.* (2002), "Sexual Mixing Patterns and Sex-Differentials in Teenage Exposure to HIV Infection in Rural Zimbabwe", *The Lancet*, Vol. 359, No. 9321, pp. 1896-1903.

Gregson, S., *et al.*, (2002), "Methods to Reduce Social Desirability Bias in Sex Surveys in Low-Development Settings: Experience in Zimbabwe", *Population Studies*, Vol. 53, No. 2, pp. 179-193.

Guennif, S., (2004), "AIDS in India: Public Health Related Aspects of Industrial and Intellectual Property Rights Policies in a Developing Country", French Research Institutes in India, Rajdhani Art Press, New Delhi.

Gupta, G.R.; (2000), "Gender, Sexuality and HIV/AIDS: The What, The Why, and The How", *http://www.gender.co.za/gendersexualityhivaids.pdf*, retrieved on 4-5-2006.

Gupta, I., Panda, S., & Motihar, R., (2003), "HIV/AIDS and Development in India", SIDA, New Delhi.

Haour-Knipe & Rector (2002), ed, "*Crossing Borders: Migration, Ethnicity and AIDS*", Taylor & Francis Ltd, London, *www. gigapedia.org*, retrieved on 4.9.2007.

Hunter, W.W., (1876), "The Statistical Account of Bengal, Districts of Darjeeling and Jalpaiguri and State of Kuch Behar", Londonif Sciences, (1987), "*Confronting AIDS: Directions for Public Health, Health Care, and Research*", National Academy Press, Washington DC, Institute of Medicine & National Academy.

International Treatment Preparedness Coalition, (2005), "Missing the Target: A Report on HIV/AIDS Treatment Access from the Frontline", Nov, Cape Town, South Africa.

Jacobson, N., (2007), "Dignity and Health: A Review", *Social Science & Medicine,* Vol. 64, No. 2, pp. 292-302.

Janssen, R.S., Holtgrave, D.R., Valdiserri, R.O., Shepherd, M., Gayle, H.D., and De Cock, K. M., (2001), "The Serostatus Approach to Fighting the HIV Epidemic: Prevention Strategies for Infected Individuals", *American Journal of Public Health,* Vol. 91, No. 7, pp. 1019-1024.

Jewkes, R.K., Levin, J., & Penn-Kekana, L., (2003), "Gender Inequalities, Intimate Partner Violence and HIV Preventive Practice: Findings of a South African Cross-Sectional Study", *Social Science & Medicine,* Vol. 56, No. 1, pp. 125-134.

Kadiyala, S., & Barneet, T., (2004), "AIDS in India: Disaster in the Making", *EPW,* May 8, pp. 1888-1892.

Kakar, D.N. and Kakar, S.N. (2001), "Combating AIDS in the 21st Century: Issues and Challenges", Sterling Publishers Private Limited, p. 32.

Kalichman, S.C., (1998), "Understanding AIDS: Advances in Research and Treatment", American Psychological Association, Washington.

Kapoor, S., (2003), "Addressing Gender Concerns in AIDS Vaccine Trials in India", *IAVI,* New Delhi.

Kauffman, C.E., Clark, S., Manzini, N., May, J., (2004), "Communities, Opportunities, and Adolescents: Behaviour in Kwa Zulu-Natal, South Africa", *Studies in Family Planning,* Vol. 35, No. 4, pp. 261-274.

Kielmann, K., (2005) "Private providers and HIV testing in Pune, India: Challenges and Opportunities", *AIDS Care,* Vol. 17, No. 6, pp. 757-766 *http://taylorandfrancis.metapress.com/(tsp4ph2iatxswb45iejuzren)/app/home/contribution.asp?referrer=parent&backto=issue,10,12;journal,7,81;linkingpublicationresults,1:100631,1*

Kingsley, L.A., Detels, R., Kaslow, R.B.F., Rinaldo, C.R., & Chieml, J., (1987), "Risk Factors for Seroconversion to Human Immunodeficiency Virus Among Male Homosexuals", *The Lancet,* Vol. 1. pp. 345-349.

Kishore, J., (2005), "National Health Programmes of India", Century Publications, New Delhi.

Leshabari S.C., Blystad, A., Moland, Km., (2007) "Difficult Choices:

Infant Feeding Experiences of HIV-Positive Mothers in Northern Tanzania", *www.sahara.org.za/index.php/Download-document/203-Difficult-choices-Infant-feeding-experiences-of-HIV-pos. retrieved on 2.1.2008*

Li. L., *et al.*, (2007), "Using Case Vignettes to Measure HIV-Related Stigma among Health Professionals in China", *International Journal of Epidemiology*, Vol. 36, No. 1, pp. 178-184.

Link, B.G., & Phelan, J.C., (2006), "Stigma and its Public Health Implications", *The Lancet*, Vol. 367, pp. 528-529.

Lorber, J., (1997), "Gender and Social Construction of Illness", Sage Publications, New Delhi.

MacDonald, D.S., (1996), "Notes on the Socio-Economic and Cultural Factors Influencing the Transmission of HIV in Botswana", *Social Science & Medicine*, Vol. 42, No. 9, pp. 1325-1333.

Mahal, A., (2004), "Economic Implications of Inertia on HIV/AIDS and Benefits of Action", *EPW*, Vol. 39, No. 10, 6 March, pp. 1049-1063.

Mahalik, J.R., Burns, S.M., Syzdek, M., (2007), "Masculinity and Perceived Normative Health Behaviours as Predictors of Men Health Behaviour", *Social Science & Medicine*, Vol. 64, No. 11, pp. 2201-2209.

Mak, W.W.S., Cheung, R.Y.M. *et al.*, (2007), "Examining Attribution Model of Self-Stigma on Social Support and Psychological Well-Being Among People with HIV+/AIDS", *Social Science & Medicine*, Vol. 64, No. 8, pp. 1549-1559.

Manderson, L., Tye, L.C., & Rajanayagam, K., (2005), "Condom Use in Heterosexual Sex: A Review of Research 1985-1994", in Catalan, J., Sherr, L., & Hedge, B., (ed), "The Impact of AIDS: Psychological and Social Aspects of HIV Infection", Taylor & Francis e-Library, Amsterdam, *www. gigapedia*.org, retrieved on 4.9.2007.

Marin, B.V., (1996), "Cultural Issues in HIV Prevention for Latinos: Should We Try to Change Gender Roles", in Oskamp, S., & Thompson, S.C. (ed), "Understanding and Preventing HIV Risk Behaviour: Safer Sex and Drug Use", Sage Publications, New Delhi.

Masanjala, W,. (2007), "The poverty-HIV/AIDS nexus in Africa: A Livelihood Approach", *Social Science & Medicine*, Vol. 64, No. 5, pp. 1032-1041.

McKee, N., Bertrand, T.J., and Benton, A.B., (2004) "Strategic Communication in the HIV/AIDS Epidemic", Sage Publications, New Delhi,.

Metha, L., (2003), "India's Creeping Plague", *Himal*, Vol. 16, No. 3, March, pp. 7-16.

Miller, C.M., *et al.*, (2007), "Emerging Health Disparities in Botswana: Examining the Situation of Orphans During the AIDS Epidemic", *Social Science and Medicine*, Vol. 64, No. 12, pp. 2476-2486.

Mitchell, A.D. and Bossert, T., (2007), "Measuring Dimensions of Social Capital: Evidence from Surveys in Poor Communities in Nicaragua", *Social Science and Medicine*, Vol. 64, No. 1, pp. 50-63.

Mondragon, D., Kirkman-Life, B., & Schneller, E.S., (1991), "Hostility to People with AIDS: Risk Perception and Demographic Factors", *Social Science and Medicine*, Vol. 32, No. 10, pp-.1137-1142.

Moore, A.R., & Oppong, J.R., (2007), "Sexual Risk Behaviour Among People Living with HIV/AIDS in Togo", *Social Science and Medicine*, Vol. 64, No. 5, pp. 1057-1066.

Munoz-Silva, A. *et al.*, (2007), "AIDS Prevention in Late Adolescent College Students from Spain and Portugal", *Public Health*, Vol. 121, No. 9, September, pp. 673-681.

Muthuswamy, V., (2005), "Ethical issues in HIV/AIDS Research", ICMR, April, New Delhi, pp. 601-610.

NACO (2004), "Annual Report 2002-03, 2003-04 (Up to July), Ministry of Health and Family Welfare, GOI, New Delhi.

NACO (2005), "UNGASS India report: Progress report on the declaration of commitment on HIV/AIDS", Ministry of Health and Family Welfare, GOI, New Delhi.

NACO, (2006), "National AIDS Control Programme: Phase III (2007-2012)", Ministry of Health and Family Welfare, GOI, New Delhi.

NACO, (2007), "HIV Facts Sheets: Based on HIV Sentinel Surveillance Data in India 2003-2006", Ministry of Health and Family Welfare, GOI, New Delhi.

Nag, M., (2001), "Anthropological Perspectives on Prostitution and AIDS in India", *EPW*, Vol. 36, No. 42, 20-26 Oct, pp. 4025-4030.

Naik, T.K., Sarkar, S., Singh, H.L., Bhunia, S.C., Singh, Y.I., Singh, P., & Pal, S.C., (1991), "Intravenous Drug Users—A New High Risk Group of HIV Infection in India."

National Institute on Alcohol Abuse and Alcoholism, "Alcohol: A

Priority for HIV/AIDS Research", (*http://www.niaaa.nih.gov/ResearchInformation/ExtramuralResearch/NIAAAResearch Areas/perspect.htm* retrieved on 7.7.2007)

Nelkin, D., Willis, D.P., Parris S.V. ed., (1991), "Cultural and Institutional Responses to AIDS", Cambridge University Press, New York.

NICED, (2006), "Studies on HIV/AIDS: Study on the Sexually Transmitted Infection Among Female Sex Workers of West Bengal", *NICED*, Annual Report 2004-2005, *http://www.niced.org*. retrieved on 11.10.2006.

Ojha, V.P., & Pradhan, B.K., (2006), "The Macro-Economic and Sectoral Impact of HIV and AIDS in India: A CGE Analysis", *http://www.undp.org.in/HIVAIDS/reports/CGE.pdf*, retrieved on 5.11.2006.

O'Malley, L.S.S. (1989), "Bengal District Gazetteers: Darjeeling", Logos Press, New Delhi.

Oppong, J., (1998), "A Vulnerability Interpretation of the Geography of HIV/AIDS in Ghana 1986-1995", *The Professional Geography*, Vol. 50, No. 4, pp. 437-448.

Oskamp, S., & Thompson, S.C. (ed), (1996), "Understanding and Preventing HIV Risk Behaviour: Safer Sex and Drug Use", Sage Publications, New Delhi.

Ow, R., & Katz, D., (1999), "Family Secrets and the Disclosure of Distressful Information in Chinese Families", *Families in Society*, Vol. 80, No. 6, pp. 620-628.

Panda, S. (2002), "The HIV/AIDS Epidemic in India: An Overview", in Panda, S., Chatterjee, A. and Abdul-Quader, A.S. (Eds.), "Living with the AIDS Virus: The Epidemic and The Response in India", Sage Publications, New Delhi, p. 20.

Panda, S., *et al.* (ed)., (2002), "Living with the AIDS Virus: The Epidemic and The Response in India," Sage Publications, New Delhi.

Panos, (1990), "Triple Jeopardy: Women & AIDS", The PANOS Institute, London.

Panos, (1999), "AIDS Reports: Investigating An Epidemic", PANOS Institute, South Asia, Nepal.

Pierret, J., (2007), "An Analysis Over Time (1990-2000) of the Experiences of Living with HIV", *Social Science & Medicine*, Vol. 65, No. 8, pp. 1595-1605.

Pinn, F., (1990), "The Road of Destiny: Darjeeling Letters 1839", Oxford University Press, Delhi.

Ramasubban, R., & Rishyasringa, B., (2005), "AIDS and Civil Society: India's Learning Curve", Rawat Publications, New Delhi.

Ramasundaram, S., (2002), "Care Without Drugs", *Seminar*, No. 520, Dec, pp. 51-52.

—— (2002), "Can India Avoid Being Devastated by HIV", *British Medical Journal*, Vol. 324, 26 January, pp. 182-183.

Rhodes, F. & Malotte, C.K., (1996), "HIV Risk Interventions for Active Drug Users: Experience and Prospects", in Oskamp, S. & Thompson S.C. ed, "Understanding and Preventing HIV Risk Behaviour: Safer Sex and Drug Use", Sage Publications, New Delhi.

Ridge, D., *et al.*, (2007), "Positive Prevention: Contemporary issues facing HIV positive people negotiating sex in the UK", *Social Science and Medicine*, Vol. 65, No. 4, pp. 755-770.

Ritu Priya, (2003), "Health Services and HIV Treatment: Complex Issues and Options", *EPW*, Vol. 38, No. 50, 13-19 Dec, pp. 5227-5232.

——, (2003), "Rethinking AIDS as Social Responsibility", Report of a workshop at the Asian Social Forum (2003) Organised collaboratively by Swasthya Panchayat-Lokayan, Centre for the Study of Developing Societies and Action Aid, India.

Sambamoorti, U. *et al.*, (2004), "Antenatal Care and AIDS Knowledge Among Married Women", *EPW*, Vol. 39, No. 7, 14-20 Feb, pp. 721-727.

Samson, C., ed, (1999), "Health Studies: A Critical and Cross Cultural Reader", Routledge, London.

Samuelson, H., (2006), "Love, Lifestyles and the Risk of AIDS: The Moral Worlds of Young People in Bobo-Dioulasso, Burkina Faso", *Culture, Health and Sexuality*, Vol. 8, No. 3, pp. 211-224.

Santhya, K.G. and Jejebhoy, S., (2007), "Early Marriage and HIV/AIDS: Risk Factors Among Young Women in India", *EPW*, Vol. 42, No. 14, 7-13 April, pp. 1291-1297.

Sarkar, S., Mookherjee, P., & Roy, A., (1991), "Descriptive Epidemiology of Intervenous Herion Users—A New Risk Group for Transmission of HIV in India", *Journal of Infection*, Vol. 23, pp. 201-207.

Sarkar, S., Das, N., Panda, S., Naik, T.K., Sarkar, K., Singh, B.C., Ralte, J.M., Aier, S.M., & Tripathy, S.P., (1994), "Rapid Spread of HIV Among Injecting Drug Users in the North Eastern States of India", *Bulletin on Narcotics*, Vol. XLV, pp. 91-105.

Scambler, G., & Higgs, P., ed (1998), "Modernity, Medicine and Health: Medical Studies Towards 2000", Routledge, London.

Seddon, D.J., (1995), "AIDS in Nepal: Issues for Consideration", *Himalayan Research Bulletin*, Vol. 15, No. 2, pp. 2-11.

Seddon, D.J., (1998), "HIV/AIDS in Nepal: The Coming Crisis", *Bulletin of Concerned Asian Scholars*, Vol. 30, No. 1, January-March, pp 35-45.

Simbayi, L.C., Kalichman, S. *et al.*, (2007), "Internalised Stigma, Discrimination, and Depression Among Men and Women Living With HIV/AIDS in Cape Town, South Africa", *Social Science & Medicine*, Vol. 64, No. 9, pp. 1823-1831.

Simpson, A., (2004), "Communication and Sex Education in Families", in Burtney, E. and Duffy, M. ed. "Young People and Sexual Health: Individual, Social and Policy Contexts", Palgrave, New York.

Singh, R., (2007), "Behavioural Changes in the Family and Community of HIV-Infected People: A Case Study of Mumbai", *Social Change*, June, Vol. 37, No. 2, pp. 1-28.

Sivaram, S. and Celentano, D.D., (2003), "Training outreach workers for AIDS prevention in rural India: Is it sustainable?" *Health Policy and Planning*, Vol. 18, No. 4, pp. 411-420.

Srinivasan, S. and Sukumar, M. (2006), "Liberalization and HIV in Kerala", Social Policy and Development Programme, Paper No. 26, April, United Nations Research Institute for Social Development, *http://www.unrisd.org* retrieved on 26.10.2006.

Standing, H., (2002), "An Overview of Changing Agendas in Health Sector Reforms", Reproductive Health Matters, www.elsevier.com/locate/rhm, retrieved on 5.6.2006

The Telegraph., (2008), "HIV Awareness Tops Minister List", April 8, *http://www.darjeelingtimes.com/news/News/India-not-ready-to-legalise-commercial-sex.html*, retrieved on 6.7.2008.

Stimson, G.V., (2005), "Drug Injecting and the Spreading of HIV Infection in South-East Asia", in Catalan, J., Sherr, L., & Hedge, B., (ed), "The Impact of AIDS: Psychological and Social Aspects of HIV Infection", Taylor & Francis e-Library, Amsterdam, *www. gigapedia.org*, retrieved on 4.9.2007.

Subba, T.B., (1992), "Ethnicity, State and Development: A Case Study of Gorkhaland Movement in Darjeeling", Har Anand Publications, New Delhi.

Sundas, B., (2004), "Alcohol Consumption and Health of the People in Darjeeling Hills: An Analysis of Socio-Cultural and Developmental Factors", Dissertation submitted to the Centre for Social Medicine and Community Health, Jawaharlal Nehru University, New Delhi.

— —(2006), "Health and health-seeking behaviour among Nepali Migrants in Delhi", Paper Presented at National Conference on Identity and Nationality of the Indian-Nepalese: Issues and Perspectives, Gangtok.

Sybylla, R., (2001), "Hearing Whose Voice? The Ethics of Care and the Practices of Liberty: A Critique", *Economy and Society*, Vol. 30, No. 1, pp. 66-84.

Thimothy, R., Rajan, S.I., (2004), "Awareness and Knowledge About HIV/AIDS in India: Evidences from RCH Survey (1998-99), *Demography India*, Vol. 33, No. 1, pp. 61-83.

Tumushabe, J., (2006), "The Politics of HIV/AIDS in Uganda", Social Policy and Development Programme Paper, No. 28, August, United Nations Research Institute for Social Development, *http://www.unrisd.org* retrieved on 26.10.2006.

Turner, J.H., (2003), "The Structure of Sociological Theory", Belmont, CA: Wadsworth.

Ulin, P.R., (1992), "African Women and AIDS: Negotiating Behavioural Change", *Social Science & Medicine*, Vol. 34, No. 1, pp. 63-73.

UNAIDS, (2007), "AIDS Epidemic Update 2007", Geneva, Switzerland.

UNAIDS, (2008), "AIDS Epidemic Update 2008", Geneva, Switzerland.

UNAIDS, (2007), "A Non-governmental Organization's National Response to HIV: The Working of the All Ukrainian Network of People Living with HIV", Geneva, Switzerland.

UNAIDS, (2003), "HIV/AIDS and Young People: Hope for Tomorrow", Geneva, Switzerland.

UNAIDS, (2005), "The 'Three Ones' in Action: Where We Are and Where We Go From Here", Geneva, Switzerland.

UNAIDS (2006), "The Road Towards Universal Access: Scaling up Access to HIV Prevention Treatment, Care and Support", *http://data.unaids.org/Topics/UniversalAccess/UniversalAccess_Concept_Jan2006_en.pdf, retrieved on 5.4.2006.*

UNAIDS, (2006), "A Conceptual Framework and Basis for Action: HIV/AIDS Stigma and Discrimination", Geneva, Switzerland.

UNAIDS, (2002) HIV and AIDS-related Discrimination, Stigmatization and Denial", Geneva, Switzerland, *http://data.unaids.org/Publications/IRC-pub02/JC650-CompAnal_en.pdf,* retrieved on 7.6.2006.

UNAIDS, (2001), "Consultation on STD Intervention for Preventing HIV: What is the Evidence?" Geneva, Switzerland.

UNAIDS (2004), "2004 Report on Global AIDS Epidemic", Geneva, Switzerland.

UNAIDS (2005), "AIDS Epidemic Update Dec 2005", Geneva, Switzerland.

UNAIDS (2010), "UNAIDS Report on the Global Aids Epidemic – 2010", http://www.unaids.org/globalreport/documents/20101123_GlobalReport_full_en.pdf. retrived on 10.06.2011.

UNDP (2003), "Socio-economic impact of HIV/AIDS in Vietnam: A Preliminary Note", *http://www.undp.org.vn/undp/docs/2003/seimpact/seimpacte.pdf*

UNDP (2004), "No Safety Signs Here: Research Study on Migration and HIV Vulnerability from Seven South and North-East Asian Countries", New Delhi.

Waal, A de (2006), "AIDS and Power: Where There is No Political Crisis-Yet", Zed Books, London.

Wainberg, M.L., Gonzalez, M.A. *et al.*, (2007), "Targeted Ethnography as a Critical Step to Inform Cultural Adaptations of HIV Prevention Interventions for Adults with Severe Mental Illness", *Social Science & Medicine,* Vol. 65, No. 2, pp. 296-308.

Wanigaratne, S., Billinton, A., & Williams, M., (2005), ed. "Initiating and Maintaining Safer Sex: Evaluation of Group Work with Gay Men", in Catalan, J., Sherr, L., & Hedge, B., (ed), "The Impact of AIDS: Psychological and Social Aspects of HIV Infection", Taylor & Francis e-Library, Amsterdam, *www.gigapedia.org,* retrieved on 4.9.2007.

Watts, C. and Kumaranauake, L., (1999), "Thinking Big, Scaling Up HIV-1 Interventions in Sub-Saharan Africa", *The Lancet,* Vol. 354, pp. 1492.

WBSAP&CS (2006), Annual Report 2005-2006, Salt Lake, Kolkata, *http://www.wbhealth.gov.in/wbsapcs/ANNUAL%20REPORT2005-06.pdf,* retrieved on 9.9. 2007.

WBSAP&CS (2007), Annual Report 2005-2006, Salt Lake, Kolkata, http://www.wbhealth.gov.in/wbsapcs/Annual%20Report-%202006-07.pdf, retrieved on 9.9. 2007.

Weiss, M.G., & Ramakrishna, J., (2006), "Stigma Interventions and Research for International Health", *The Lancet*, Vol. 367, pp. 536-538.

Welbourn A., Paxton S., (2004), "Harnessing the experiences of HIV-positive people in a positive global response to the pandemic", *Int Conf AIDS*. Jul 11-16; 15: abstract no. D11205. *http://gateway.nlm.nih.gov/MeetingAbstracts/ma?f=102277944.html*, retrieved on 3.4.2007.

Wierson, M.H., & Bright, J.L. ed. (1996), "Educational Policy, Adolescent Knowledge of HIV Risk and Sexual Behaviour in Zimbabwe and the United States", in Oskamp. S. & Thompson, S.C. ed. "Understanding and Preventing HIV Risk Behaviour: Safer Sex and Drug Use", Sage Publications, New Delhi.

Wood, K., Lambert, H., Jewkes, R., (2007), "Showing Roughness in a Beautiful Way: Talk About Love, Coercion, and Rape in South African Youth Sexual Culture", *Medical Anthropology Quarterly*, Vol. 23, No. 3, pp. 277-300.

World Bank, (2004), "HIV/AIDS Treatment and Prevention in India: Modelling the Cost and Consequences", Washington DC.

Yardley, L., ed. (1997), "*Material Discourse of Health and Illness*", Routledge, London.

Yip, W., Subramanian, S.V., *et al.* (2007), "Does Social Capital Enhance Health and Well-Being? Evidences from Rural China", *Social Science and Medicine*, Vol. 64, No. 1, pp. 35-49.

Young, I., (2004), "Exploring the Role of Schools in Sexual Health Promotion", in Burtney, E. and Duffy, M. ed. "Young People and Sexual Health: Individual, Social and Policy Contexts", Palgrave, New York.

Zachariah, A., (2006), "Access to Health Care For All: What can we Learn from the AIDS Movement", *EPW*, Vol. 41, No. 25, 24-29 June, pp. 2522-24.

Zhou, Y.R., (2007), "If You Get AIDS....You Have to Endure It Alone: Understanding the Social Construction of HIV/AIDS in China", *Social Science & Medicine*, Vol. 65, No. 2, pp. 284-295.

'Ma Pani Ta Mancha Ho,' www.darjeelingtimes.com, retrieved on 2.4.2008.

"Teen Scare", *www.darjeelingtimes.com*, retrieved on 7.5.2008.

Index